How to Grow a Healthy Human

How powerful to know that you can do something to make your future children healthier. Dr. Allison has packed this book with strategies on how you can do that.

—Dr. Josh Axe, DC, DNM, CNS,
Author of *Ancient Remedies*

Preparing the place your baby will be grown in is not only empowering, it is creating the legacy of your child's health. This is an excellent resource for real health solutions in a toxic world.

—Dr. Daniel Pompa, DPSc,
Author of *Beyond Fasting*

With millions of families facing difficulties with fertility as well as the growing number of children in the US being born with, or developing chronic health conditions, I can't stress enough the importance of what Dr. Allison is teaching in this book! With the power of chiropractic and the principles Dr. Allison discusses in this book, my wife who was diagnosed "infertile" now has her fourth in the oven.

—Dr. Dale Brown, DC,
"The Wild Doc"

In this age where information abounds, it is surprising how little is known about a woman's cycle. Just being able to appropriately track it, is new to some. Dr. Allison has brought an exciting awareness to the idea that a healthy baby, pregnancy, and postpartum period starts with the "Prep-work." This book is full of real answers to some of today's hard health problems.

—Dr. Tabatha Barber, DO, FACOOG, NCMP, IFMCP

It is great to have information in the toolbox of hormones and preparing your body for pregnancy, not only for mom, but also for the most optimal development of your bundle of joy! Dr. Allison offers great support to help you understand the intricacies, complications, and exciting challenges and changes that occur before, during, and after pregnancy. It always helps to know you are not alone in creating a plan for you and your family's future, and Dr. Allison helps create this plan.

—Dr. Deborah Rice, ND, MPH, Assistant Medical Director at Precision Analytical Laboratory

Raising a healthy human is one of the most important jobs we have. This book is a gift to anyone starting a family to not only understand the physical aspects of a mother and baby's health but also the emotional aspects. We change when we become mothers; we change the moment we realize we are going to bring life into this world. Give yourself this opportunity to help your transition into this important time in your life be as smooth and supported as possible.

—Dr. Sonya Jensen ND,
Author of *Woman Unleashed*

HOW TO GROW
A HEALTHY HUMAN

HOW TO GROW A HEALTHY HUMAN

A Foundational Guide to Prepare Your Body for Pregnancy,
Give Your Children the Healthiest Start,
and Be the Mama You Were Meant to Be

DR. ALLISON EDMONDS

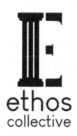

ethos
collective

How to Grow a Healthy Human © 2021 by Dr. Allison Edmonds.
All rights reserved.

Printed in the United States of America

Published by Ethos Collective™
PO Box 43, Powell, OH 43065
EthosCollective.vip

All rights reserved. This book contains material protected under international and federal copyright laws and treaties. Any unauthorized reprint or use of this material is prohibited. No part of this book may be reproduced or transmitted in any form or by any means, electronic or mechanical, including photocopying, recording, or by any information storage and retrieval system, without express written permission from the author.

LCCN: 2021913575

Paperback ISBN: 978-1-63680-053-0
Hardcover ISBN: 978-1-63680-054-7
e-book ISBN: 978-1-63680-055-4

Available in paperback, hardcover, e-book, and audiobook

Any internet addresses (websites, blogs, etc.) and telephone numbers printed in this book are offered as a resource. They are not intended in any way to be or imply an endorsement by Ethos Collective™, nor does Ethos Collective™ vouch for the content of these sites and numbers for the life of this book.

Some names and identifying details have been changed to protect the privacy of individuals.

DEDICATION

To the little dude on the front cover:
Titus, you are my favorite part about life, and you fuel my passion for the health of this next generation. When you know that God has given you a dream or tells you to do something, don't ask questions or try to make sense of it—just do the best you can every day!

> You never know how far reaching something you think,
> say, or do today will affect the lives
> of millions tomorrow.
> —B. J. Palmer

CONTENTS

Foreword................................... xi
Acknowledgments............................ xv
Introduction............................... xvii

SECTION 1: Preparing to Grow a Human........ 1

Chapter 1: You Are Your Baby's Environment....... 3

**SECTION 2: Protecting Yourself
from Inflammation and Toxins**................. 15

Chapter 2: Inflammation Is Bigger Than
         We Thought...................... 17

Chapter 3: What Are Toxins Really Affecting?..... 52

SECTION 3: Aiming for Optimal Health......... 65

Chapter 4: Are You Healthy Enough
         to Grow a Human?................ 67

Chapter 5: Repairing Your Foundation 75
Chapter 6: Removing Toxins from Your Life 106
Chapter 7: The Most Important Thing 124

Resources for the Mama-To-Be. 131
Bibliography 135
About The Author. 145

FOREWORD

We live in the most toxic time in history, and the human body is suffering because of it. Each generation is getting sicker and sicker. Chronic disease, learning disabilities, cancers, severe food allergies, and mood disorders are becoming the norm for our children. Twenty-five percent of our children are on a medication that they will take for life. This is not okay. It is time for us to panic. We have hit the tipping point where we need to do better for our children. We must ask ourselves, what is happening? Why are our children so sick? And most importantly, what can we do about it?

A decade ago, Ken Cook, CEO of the Environmental Working Group, in his talk *10 Americans* opened our eyes to the harsh reality that our children are entering this world with over two hundred chemicals already inside their bodies. We used to think that the placenta protected a child from these toxic chemicals, but evidence now reveals to us that industrial pollution begins in the womb. Because of this womb pollution, our children start life at a deficit. They are acquiring the elements of disease before they even step foot on this earth. Perhaps the most disturbing, though, is that 134 of these womb chemicals are known to cause cancer, 150 are associated with birth defects, 154 are known hormone disrupters, 186 cause infertility, 130 are immune system toxicants, and 158 are neurotoxins known to have profound effects on brain development. According to the peer reviewed medical journal *The Lancet*, "This combined evidence suggests that neurodevelopmental disorders caused by industrial chemicals has created a silent pandemic in modern society."

For our children to thrive, this reality must change. But change will not happen once they are born. Change needs to happen before a child is born. A change that needs to start with teaching women how to grow healthy humans, free from this toxic burden. How will we do this? Not only are toxins a depressing topic, but they are ubiquitous in our environment. How can we tackle this problem? Where does it start? It all starts with awareness. Awareness around what toxins we need to avoid and how we can detox them out. A detox that should take place before conception.

Finally, we have a book that teaches us how to do this. In this book, Dr. Allison Edmonds beautifully lays out for us which toxins we need to avoid and how we can properly remove these toxins from our bodies so that the next generation can live a healthy life. In the functional medicine world we have a saying called "live it to lead it." This is the idea that if you are going to lead others to a new place of health, you must have traveled the journey yourself. No one exemplifies this concept better than Dr. Edmonds. Not only has she been on a journey of detoxing herself and her family, but every day she is in the health trenches teaching couples how they can grow healthy humans and raise toxin-free kids. We need more health leaders like Dr. Edmonds!

On the pages of this book you will learn exactly which toxins you need to keep an eye out for. You will also discover alternative products you can replace these toxins with. These two steps alone will make a huge dent in your child's toxic load! But, Dr. Edmonds didn't stop there. She will walk you through different protocols to effectively detox these chemicals out of you before you get pregnant. There has never been a book written like this one and the world so desperately needs this information. When Dr. Edmonds first told me about the title of this book, I was beyond thrilled to know that a book like this would be available for couples beginning their family journey. Too many families are struggling as their children's health declines, struggles that could have possibly been avoided if this information had gotten into their hands before their children were born.

This book will save lives. No matter where you are on your family planning journey, you will benefit from the information Dr. Edmonds so eloquently lays out for us here. For those of you who already have children, no mommy guilt here. As we know better, we do better, for the health of our families. If you are thinking about getting pregnant, this could be the most important book will read on pregnancy. Let the words on these pages motivate, inspire, and empower you to move into action. Knowledge is power and when you know how to grow a healthy human, you move from being a victim of this modern world, to a champion of your child's health. We are all in this together. Our children need us now more than ever and Dr. Edmonds has given us the resources to change the fate of our children and start growing healthy humans again.

Dr. Mindy Pelz, DC
Best Selling Author of *The Reset Factor*,
The Reset Factor Kitchen, and *The Menopause Reset*
San Jose, California

ACKNOWLEDGMENTS

Several years ago the thought *I think I could write a book* popped into my head. Not long after, my mom handed me a notebook with an inspiring title she had written on the front, feeding my original thought. Just thinking of all the situations that fell perfectly into place (even if they didn't seem perfect at the time) and all the people that have encouraged, supported, and prayed for me on this journey overwhelms me with gratitude. Building a wellness center, being a full-time mom, and trying to manage all that life throws at me, I truly know God gave me the strength, energy, and the words to put into this book.

Personally, I could not have done this without my family, my parents' encouragement, and their keeping Titus our firstborn, for sleepovers so I could have a few mornings to myself. Thanks, NanNee-Bop. My father-in-law Pop-Pop, for driving in from Pennsylvania to spend several weeks so I could buckle down and just write. Julie, your prayers did more than you know! Jennie and Lauren, you helped me make sense of my thoughts when I got stuck. Cathy, holding down the office fort and helping me protect my time was essential. Oh, and my husband Daniel . . . Honey, you never looked so good as when you did the dishes, made dinner, and took care of our kid. I praise your multi-tasking skills. :) Most of all, thank you for your patience and love, even when I stress out and ride the hot-mess-express train!

Thank you to Dr. Pompa, and my whole Platinum family for pouring into me so I can be my best self, and pass on life changing information to the world. Every professional that shared their time and expertise for interviews was essential to getting this book's message out. Andrea, your coaching and prayers helped make this all happen!

I feel so blessed by all the people that have been part of this journey. This book truly is a conglomeration of all the mentors, seminars, professors, doctors, and experience with patients. Thank you, and may you use this book as a tool to bring health to your families for generations to come!

INTRODUCTION

This book is for all my Type A friends who live to plan, for the wannabe planners, and of course, anyone who wants to grow a healthy human. It is getting harder and harder to stay healthy, and the more we learn about health, the more we realize that we, and our kids, are fighting an uphill battle. The more you detox your body and home *before* growing a human, the better chance they have of living an optimally healthy life. The principles and strategies you will learn apply not only to women in their child-bearing years but also to anyone influencing or teaching young women about their bodies and cycles. Misinformation is creating a crisis of devastating health conditions that afflict people of all ages, so let's take our children's health into our own hands, and we might just improve our own health along the way.

I always value knowing who I am learning from, so I've included the shortest version of my last two decades that I could muster. I finished my undergraduate studies, went to chiropractic school, trained in an office, got married, started a practice, built it, then decided, "Okay, it's time to start a family!" I went to a seminar where Dr. Dan Pompa spoke about toxins, how they are passed down for generations, and how they shape the health of our future children, so I paused the baby idea until I could detox my body properly. I poured thousands of hours and dollars into learning everything I could about hormones, toxins, and health and healing. I implemented many of the strategies you will read about, got pregnant, and today my little dude is two and a half years old. I write this as I prepare my body a second time to grow a healthy human.

I participate in a network of doctors involved in Health Centers of the Future. I consider it a great privilege to rub elbows with so many talented doctors who truly serve as world changers. We are a unique group of doctors from many areas of medicine, and thanks to technology, we are able to collaborate on a daily basis. Collaboration makes doctors better, both as healers and as people. I am excited to share my interviews with several of these doctors; they have contributed much of the knowledge in this book.

SECTION 1
PREPARING TO GROW A HUMAN

CHAPTER 1
YOU ARE YOUR BABY'S ENVIRONMENT

What a beautiful opportunity we have to participate in the creation of another life! The blessing that God gives a woman, to play such an integral part in shaping a human life, gives me goosebumps every time I think about it. Whether you have had children or are thinking about having them, just pause for a minute and acknowledge how amazingly He created you. Not only does your body have the capacity to incubate a human as it develops, it makes adjustments to feed, sustain, and support the tiny human. When a baby's immune system is challenged, their saliva changes, and tiny receptors on the mother's nipple detect this change. In turn, they signal the mother's body to produce more antibodies. The baby relies on the mother for immune support for the first six months of life. Despite years of research on breast milk, scientists are still discovering new components, as well as the unparalleled benefits to human babies from their mother's milk compared to conventional formulas. Because of this beautiful process that is built inside of us, I always encourage mamas that cannot nurse to seek out donor milk.

Some aspects of growing a human happen automatically; the sperm meets the egg, cells divide, organs form, and a tiny brain and personality begin to develop. It is truly mind blowing when you let it all sink in. But other aspects take work. Some of you will need to change your diet, detox your body, break bad habits, condition or strengthen your body, and read and learn about the obstacles to making healthy decisions for your children. Most of these are chemical or physical, but I would argue that for true healing, we must address emotional aspects too. After all, we are all emotional beings, whether we admit it or not.

To do this, let's begin by considering the one in thirty-three babies born with a birth defect, one in fifty-nine identified as landing on the autism spectrum with numbers climbing exponentially, and numerous others who are hit with second-leading cause of death in children under age fifteen: cancer. As harsh as that might sound, I don't mean to incite fear, but to offer an understanding of the challenges we face. Our mothers and certainly our grandmothers did not have to have this conversation, but here and now we live in a different world, and we need to talk about it if we want to grow healthy humans. One powerful study explains a bit more about these obstacles and their connection to growing a healthy human.

> We live in a different world than our mothers and grandmothers, and we need to talk about the challenges we face if we want to grow healthy humans.

The Environmental Working Group examined the umbilical cord blood of newborns and found that they began life exposed to as many as 287 chemicals. In the study, an average of 200 toxins were found per baby, and 180 of those chemicals are known to cause cancer. Cancer rates in children have risen 67.1 percent since 1950, and the Columbia University School of Public Health links the cause of 95 percent of cancer to diet and the environment.

When you're growing a human, you are that environment. This, my friends, is exactly why I am writing this book and probably why you are reading it. If all those toxins exist in the cord blood, they exist in your baby, and only cleaning them out of your system will keep them from entering your baby. Check out the YouTube video "10 Americans" for a sharable visual of the study.

A well-respected doctor whose lectures I have had the pleasure of hearing several times once said, "Why would you put a bun in the oven if the oven is broken?" (Thanks, Billy D.) Whether you think your oven is broken or not, it's imperative that you address the toxins in your baby-to-be's environment if your goal is to grow a healthy human.

The Hormone Dance

When I was six weeks pregnant with my son, nausea hit me right after I ate a substantial amount of gluten-free pizza. Three-and-a-half years later, I still cannot smell that pizza without nearly tossing my cookies. The vomiting lasted several hours that night, even though I had accounted for every ingredient. Thinking it might have just been the pizza, imagine my surprise when I awoke the next morning feeling just as bad as the day before. I could barely move let alone work. Every night I went to bed thinking, *Oh, I'll feel better in the morning*, and every day I was wrong. Hello *Groundhog Day*. It really amazes me that some people feel better during pregnancy, while others have it worse than I did. Thinking there was light at the end of the first trimester tunnel, I felt equally disappointed as I spent my summer family vacation moving from the chair to the couch to lying in the boat. I was so miserable! Eventually I could work a little bit here and there, but overall, it was terrible. I tried anything and everything people suggested. I honestly remember feeling decent from week twenty-four to week twenty-eight, and that was about it. Whenever I consulted an expert, I heard the same thing—"Yep, it's your hormones. We don't know why you feel like this. It's just different for everyone."

I carried that little rascal forty-four weeks, obviously not the normal time frame. I eventually went into labor on my own, but I welcomed my healthy ten-pound baby via cesarian section. Although I don't know that I was depressed, I experienced anxiety so severe over the next four months that I would do anything to never feel that way again. All the while my doctors blamed hormones, and thus began my mission to fix them. I later learned that my *pre*-pregnancy hormones caused the difficult labor and delivery, as well as my postpartum struggles. That really gave me hope—I knew I could change things for the better the next time around.

Humans are complex beings, especially the ones who are built to reproduce.

Look at the hormone dance of a normal menstrual cycle. We know that chemical, physical, and emotional factors play into the regularity of a woman's monthly cycle. For example, if you experience high stress in the second half of your cycle (emotional, chemical, or physical), it may prolong the Luteal phase, causing your period to begin late. Understand that no matter how off-balance your cycle, it still gives you valuable information, and a great opportunity to listen to your body. Let's clarify *normal*. Normal is a twenty-eight- to thirty-three-day cycle with minimal cramping and mood swings, and bright red blood with a manageable flow.

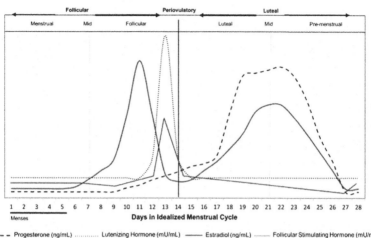

Source: Springer Nature

If your cycle is not normal, seek testing and incorporate the healing strategies discussed later in this book. Do this *before* you grow your human. Testing can be helpful, but it also can be misleading if you do not perform the right test at the precise time in your cycle. And, if you cycle irregularly—good luck getting accurate results with simple bloodwork. For example, your bloodwork may look normal, yet from our definition of a normal period, you know that it is not accurate. Saliva is another way to test hormones and although helpful for some information it also can be a misrepresentation of what is going on throughout the entire month of your cycle. I have found the best way to test your hormones is a dried urine test that you have up to five samples within a twenty-four-hour period. There are a few, but I prefer the Dutch Complete by Precision Analytical Labs. This test

> Humans are complex beings, especially the ones who are built to reproduce.

will not only give you a breakdown of each hormone and its derivatives, but also detail your cortisol and cortisone levels, yielding valuable information about your adrenals.

Dr. Debbie Rice is the assistant medical director with Precision Labs. Daily, she helps interpret the results of the highly complex Dutch hormone tests for practitioners. I gained so much valuable information from her presentation "Hormones, Pregnancy, and Postpartum." In it, she refers to the three months prior to pregnancy as *trimester zero*, the nine months of pregnancy as their usual trimesters one through three, and the three months after delivery as the *fourth trimester*. She explained that the state our hormones pre-pregnancy determines our postpartum experience. The amazing process of pregnancy requires so much energy that it is important to consider your body's readiness to handle it. We don't just want to survive it, and we don't want to be out of commission as soon as our little bundle of joy arrives. Dr. Rice explained that my zero trimester dictated my fourth trimester: I evidenced an imbalance from the beginning. Since hormones play a huge role in pregnancy, delivery, and the postpartum period, I decided to test and work on balancing mine *before* I got pregnant again.

This entire book centers around trimester zero. In light of understanding the complexity of our hormones in pregnancy, I will now break down their changes as an egg gets fertilized. No quiz will follow this section, so just soak up as much information as you can.

Here's what happens to your hormones when you become pregnant:

- Estrogen stimulates ovulation and builds up the endometrium.
- Progesterone aids in implanting the egg into the endometrium and tells the body to stop menstruation.

- HCG supports the development of the egg inside the ovary and supports progesterone production until the placenta is formed. It also helps form the placenta once implantation occurs.

- During the first trimester, estrogen climbs to help signal organ development in the baby. Progesterone aids in protecting the endometrial lining to help reduce rejection of the embryo, and it suppresses uterine contractions.

- HCG saves the corpus luteum from involuting or shriveling up so it can continue to make progesterone. Around eight to nine weeks of gestation, the placenta takes over the production of progesterone.

The baby continues to develop for the remaining thirty-eight to forty-two weeks, and then its birth time arrives. Do you know that the baby initiates hormone signals to the mama? It all starts in their tiny little brains, or more specifically their hypothalamic pituitary adrenal communication, or HPA axis. Their body releases cortisol that causes the mom's uterus to up-regulate more oxytocin receptors, which causes a drop in progesterone, allowing for estrogen dominance (remember progesterone was preventing uterine contractions.) As the estrogen dominates, it sets off a release of prostaglandins to help increase uterine contractions so mom can push that baby out!

After estrogen and progesterone give their all in the delivery, they crash. The fourth trimester, six to twelve weeks post-delivery, basically mimics menopause. Here, a woman relies on oxytocin. It helps us love our baby and reminds us that labor was not only worth it, but what our bodies were made for. It comes in waves while we nurse, and some women report feeling a constant natural high for up to two weeks. In the presence of additional stress or inflammation, however, cortisol that would normally convert to serotonin, contributing to those positive feelings, instead converts to another substance that causes oxidative stress.

So there's good news and bad news. The good news is you don't have to remember any of that for your body to do what it was created to do. God programmed the symphony of hormones in you, and all you need to do is readily listen to your body when the time comes. The bad news? If your health is inadequate, and you fail to listen to and support your body in this amazing process, you will have a rough recovery, and sadly others will suffer with you. Stay tuned for supportive strategies to stay healthy while you grow a healthy human!

PCOS, Endometriosis, Fibroids, and Irregular Periods

Through the complexity of the last few paragraphs, I intended to create a state of awe for how amazingly God created our bodies. But what if imbalanced hormones are your reality right now? In the case of PCOS or Polycystic Ovarian Syndrome, your ovaries may be developing fluid filled cysts that will interfere with your ability to ovulate properly, and therefore make it difficult to conceive. PCOS sufferers also experience irregular periods, acne, and even abnormal facial or body hair while losing hair on the head. PCOS treatment sometimes involves the same medications used to treat diabetes, because of the intimate relationship between our sex hormones and insulin.

Endometriosis is a chronic, inflammatory, hormone-dependent disease where endometrial tissue grows outside the uterus. Current research shows that cruciferous vegetables aid the immune system decreasing the symptoms and severity of endometriosis. Fibroids are non-cancerous growths that develop in the uterus. At one point, scientists thought that estrogen drove fibroids and other conditions of the uterus, but additional research demonstrates that inflammation, rather than estrogen or progesterone, negatively affects the hormone dance occurring every month in our bodies.

Whatever your hormonal challenges, your doctors might have told you that you would never get pregnant, or that you would have to take medication for the rest of your life and hope it would enable you to carry a tiny human. Or maybe "Dr. Google" helped diagnose you, and the more you read, the more devastated you became. Or possibly you are reading this thinking your cycle is perfect because you have been taking a birth control for so long you have no idea what your period would be like without it.

I would like to challenge whatever your reality is right now. What if we could find the reason behind your hormone imbalance? What if we could get to the root cause and begin reducing inflammation and initiate healing your body? Rarely does an estrogen problem or hormone deficiency alone cause pregnancy problems. Instead, we must consider a balance of all the hormones and their interactions. This is really great news as it puts the ball back in our court, so to speak. We know how to decrease inflammation, which in turn will optimize our insulin sensitivity, which directly relates to all of our sex hormones.

If you fall into one of the categories above with a hormonal challenge, I am confident by the end of this book, you will better understand how your condition might have developed and what to do about it. In this day and age, one in eight couples cannot conceive. If you have been there, you know firsthand the serious difficulty of navigating this situation, which unfortunately is expected to worsen in the next generation. If you have not been able

> Rarely does an estrogen problem or hormone deficiency alone cause pregnancy problems. Instead, we must consider a balance of all the hormones and their interactions.

to conceive with or without intervention, or if you have had one or multiple miscarriages, there is still hope! If we know that inflammation underlies hormone dysfunction, and toxins contribute most largely to inflammation, why not eliminate the culprit, incorporate more supportive habits, and let your body heal to do what it was designed to do—grow a healthy human.

A Note about Miscarriages

If you or someone close to you has had one or multiple miscarriages, you know all too well the emotional and physical difficulty involved. I hope the previous discussion about the body's intricate hormone dance will bring peace and solace to those who felt they might have somehow caused their miscarriage. I certainly felt better after learning these concepts, and I will talk more about my personal experience in this section.

Good friends of mine had a miscarriage around eight to ten weeks of gestation. They had already received a seemingly healthy ultrasound picture, told the family they were expecting, and prepared their excited two-year-old daughter for being a big sister. Then the pain started. Cramping and spotting took them to the hospital, where they discovered the baby was no longer alive. Scheduled for a D&C (It stands for dilation and curettage) several days later, faced with telling family, and feeling deep sorrow, my friend was in a rough place. She wondered if she would be able to carry another child and started racking her brain for any mistakes she made. If you have experienced a miscarriage, you can relate to her experience, so you might be equally justified in your anger as I tell you the next part. Her mother-in-law (probably wanting to check on her and distract her from the pain) brought a friend over to boast about her garden, perhaps hoping that would cheer her up. Apparently to clear the elephant from the room, she quickly announced upon the woman's arrival, "Well, Haley lost her baby." Needless to say, my friend had to leave the room. It hurt her in so many ways.

A few years later, after having my own experience of a very painful miscarriage, I think I understand something new about dealing with the aftermath of a miscarriage. I *hate* to lose things. I am hard on myself if I lose a file or a key or anything else insignificant. I literally cannot let it go until I find it. So the first time I heard someone say, "Oh, Allison lost her baby," I flipped out. I most certainly did not lose anything! After I wrestled with the truth of whether I really lost a baby, I began to not only instantly change the way I spoke about miscarriage, but to reshape the way I thought about it and sought to teach others.

Someone that was inside of me is now gone. A person growing inside of me, and the profound awareness of this made me constantly feel like I was forgetting something or something was missing. I share this because I believe in the importance of our experiences, and I believe that we can honor them by speaking truth over them. We know that a miscarriage naturally occurs when a sperm and an egg don't properly unite to become a grown human. But no matter how much you know intellectually, you still have to process the emotional experience of a miscarriage.

> No matter how much you know intellectually, you still have to process the emotional experience of a miscarriage.

With advanced technology and research, we now know that vaccines and environmental factors play the largest role in increased miscarriage rates. One in four pregnancies result in miscarriage, and it is all too easy to just brush over the statistics, which is why I shared my friend's story. One in four reflects a major problem and constitutes one of the primary reasons I wanted to write this book.

I know that having a miscarriage enabled me to have compassion and empathy for others struggling with this experience; it was a part of my own beautiful journey. There was nothing I could do about it. I didn't do anything wrong. Moving forward, I hope to decrease the chances of it happening again by strengthening my body through all the great strategies in this book. At the end of the day, I find peace in knowing that even when I don't understand why, the Bible tells me in Jeremiah 29:11 that God has a plan to give me hope and a good future. I believe this with my whole heart, so after allowing myself to feel all my emotions and honor the experience, I chose not to settle in despair. Instead, I file it in the "moving on even when I don't understand" space, and do just that.

SECTION 2
PROTECTING YOURSELF FROM INFLAMMATION AND TOXINS

CHAPTER 2
INFLAMMATION IS BIGGER THAN WE THOUGHT

We know hormones are important in growing a human, but we also need the rest of our body in balance as well. Now that we have different doctors for our kidneys, heart, gut, and "Oh, you have a problem with your hair falling out? You need a thyroid doctor." We start to think organ systems of our body operate separately from one another. Not true, of course, but to treat people wholistically, we need to view all the interactions of our bodies' systems to create balance and homeostasis. We also need to look for the root causes of disorder, such as the under-functioning of one system or the hyperactivity of another.

Time Magazine's stellar cover story on inflammation as "The Secret Killer" connected cancer, heart disease, Alzheimer's, and other diseases linked to inflammation. Hardly a day goes by without a new publication about inflammation and how it underlies chronic disease.

Inflammation is a natural protective process that protects our bodies from infections, injuries, and toxins. We easily understand inflammation with an ankle sprain. The ankle swells up and turns red as the body delivers more blood and nutrients to the area. All the while the swelling actually acts as a splint to protect your ankle while it heals. When you encounter a virus or bacteria, your body temperature goes up to fight off the invader and starts a cascade of inflammatory reactions that help the body to heal—then the inflammation shuts down. But what happens when you encounter invaders that alter the way your immune system functions? Things like heavy metals, physical and emotional trauma, and thousands of toxic chemicals we encounter every day can stress our bodies into a state of chronic inflammation. This inflammation occurs at a cellular level and affects the tiny, intricate functions of our cells, tissues, and organ systems. Research findings, for example, demonstrate that patients on anti-inflammatory medications experience fewer heart attacks than normally expected. Now, I am *not* telling you to take anti-inflammatory drugs to prevent heart attacks! I *am* saying that if decreasing inflammation can prevent disease, why would we not do everything in our power to understand inflammation and eliminate it? *Ooh-whee!* I get excited as the puzzle comes together: *toxins = inflammation = dis-ease and dysfunction.*

> If decreasing inflammation can prevent disease, why would we not do everything in our power to understand inflammation and eliminate it?

INFLAMMATION IS BIGGER THAN WE THOUGHT

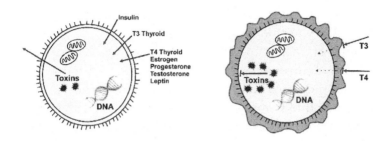

Take note of the picture on the left. This is a normal healthy cell, with a membrane made of a phospholipid bilayer. It allows nutrients to flow inside easily, and toxins and free radicals to exit the cell. Each of the hormones listed has to bind to a receptor on the cell membrane to get its message in the cell. This signals each cell to carry out its unique function.

Now take note of the second picture on the right. This is an inflamed membrane in a person exposed to toxins such as chemicals or harmful fats. The membrane becomes inflamed because toxins are stored in fats. This blocks the receptors from connecting to important hormones and nutrients that need to enter the cell. The inflamed membrane does not allow toxins to exit the cell, so it becomes sick, inflamed, and cannot function properly. The toxins trapped inside the cell also damage its DNA by turning on wrong codes or turning off the right ones. This process significantly weighs into the understanding of all chronic diseases.

It explains why someone with "normal" blood work may not feel well. Their hormones may be within normal ranges within the blood, but if the hormone cannot bind to cell receptors, they cannot get their message into the cell. When testing looks normal, doctors tell you you're fine. However, their extracellular blood work doesn't indicate if hormonal messages are getting inside the cells. This, my friends, shows why you can have a legitimate hormone imbalance, thyroid problem, weight loss problem, or more, even when your blood work looks normal.

Since fat makes up membranes, let's evaluate the quality of fats you consume. Good fats, important for more than just your new keto diet, keep your cell membranes healthy, translating into many health benefits. Bad fats will damage the membrane faster than good fats can heal it. If you eat out at restaurants, you consume bad fats, as vegetable oil, corn oil, canola/rapeseed oil, and peanut oil are the most cost-effective oils for a restaurant to use. Unfortunately for us, manufacturers process these oils to the point that they become rancid, creating inflammation in both the outer membrane of the cell but also inner membranes like those that surround our mitochondria. Mitochondria serve as our little energy factories, so we don't want those malfunctioning whether we are trying to grow a human or not. Bottom line, bad fats do more than just make you fat; they affect you at a cellular level and mess with your hormones.

> Bad fats do more than just make you fat; they affect you at a cellular level and mess with your hormones.

Consequences of Inflammation

Dr. Dan Pompa is a global leader and expert in detoxing and reducing inflammation at a cellular level. He created the True Cellular Detox program, and through a multi-therapeutic approach, has helped thousands of seriously ill people recover their health. He stated, "I believe there are three main toxins affecting four generations that are leading to an explosion of chronic diseases and unexplainable illnesses. And those three toxins are mercury, lead, and aluminum." I chose Dr. Pompa as a mentor in part because he served on the front lines, training other doctors to detox children after the lead crisis in Flint, Michigan. Together with my platinum team of docs, we truly lead the world in proper detoxification protocols. I will share our personal experience with toxins and specifically how you can stop or even reverse the damage from them, so you can prepare the best environment for your future kiddos.

The CDC says that six out of ten Americans have at least one chronic condition and four out of ten have multiple. It goes on to name the key contributing factors as tobacco use, inactivity, poor nutrition, and alcohol abuse. How many people do you know that don't feel well, can't get pregnant, or have sick kids, yet they don't engage in any of those behaviors? We know a deeper cause underlies this health crisis. In 2009, *The Lancet* published an article stating that 80 percent of disease could be eliminated with preventative changes like diet and exercise. However, every day people come to our office, tired of being sick, and they say, "I don't drink or smoke, I exercise, and I eat organic, so why am I still sick?" or "Why can't I function without these medications?" Seventy-eight percent of all Americans over 55 have at least one chronic disease. We're talking truly debilitating issues including diabetes, heart disease, cancer, thyroid dysfunction, digestive disorders, irritable bowel syndrome (IBS), Crohn's disease, inflammatory conditions, joint conditions, immune dysfunction, and autoimmune conditions. As I get closer to fifty-five years of age, that number looks younger and younger. And we know that if you're diagnosed with one condition, you're more likely to have multiple. By the time you show symptoms of a disorder, the organ system involved has been stressed for at least ten years. We can then estimate that it only functions at a fraction of its capacity. You don't want your car functioning around 60 percent, do you? No, and you can't have quality of life at half your body's normal level of functioning. When you experience symptoms such as headaches, neck or back pain, chronic infections, and fatigue, they tell us that your system has been breaking down for years. I'm excited to give you tools for yourself or your family to recover your health, because we know that toxins form the root of literally every disease. We now know that environmental factors cause over 90 percent of diseases. In fact, Dr. Bruce Lipton, referred to as "The Father of Epigenetics," states that genetics cause only *1 percent* of disease.

> By the time you show symptoms of a disorder, the organ system involved has been stressed for at least ten years.

Our health has come to such a devastating place that it seems the main topic of conversation for people. At my last family reunion, I took a mental survey of the number of conversations that centered on health conditions. I had an easier time counting the conversations that did not center around their health as literally it seemed that it is all people talked about. I thought people raised the issue with me because they know I am a doctor, but actually people regularly discuss it. They talk about it at work, on the phone, and with their friends, and you can't turn on the TV or radio without hearing about a drug, health condition, or a lawsuit from a drug or exposure. And the prayer list at church—cancer, fibromyalgia, surgery. We are all falling apart, and I do not believe God intended this for us. These conditions are not a natural part of aging. Now that we know the role that inflammation and toxins play, we can start to take action.

It's also important to talk about the diseases and medical conditions on the rise in our children. Dr. Stephanie Seneff predicts that on the present scale of growth, by 2032, one out of every two children in the United States and 80 percent of boys will land on the autism spectrum. Dr. Seneff has published a phenomenal amount of research on this topic, and I highly recommend her resources. While an emotionally charged topic, most doctors agree that autism results from many factors, but the basis of the discussion returns to toxins and the child's ability to properly detoxify.

According to the CDC, diabetes will basically become an epidemic, with one in every three children born after the year 2000 developing diabetes in his or her lifetime. Diabetes is a condition of insulin resistance, and insulin resistance causes hormonal imbalances, neurological problems, weight problems, and many other conditions. So it is not just the diabetes that is a problem, it's the other dysfunctions that will occur secondary to the condition.

Sadly, diabetes is not our only concern. According to the American Cancer Society's *Cancer Facts & Figures 2021*, cancer has become the second most common cause of death, exceeded only by heart disease. That report also states that more than 1,670 Americans will die per day from cancer (not just adults, but our children, totaling 608,570 people in the year 2021). Cancer rates in children have risen 67.1 percent since 1950. And according to Columbia University's School of Public Health, *diet and environment* cause 95 percent of cancer. The toxin load of children at birth and what they cumulatively gain over time also contributes to the picture. I guarantee that cancer has touched every person reading this book, whether through a grandparent, a cousin, or another, but now we see younger and younger children plagued with it. I know these things are hard to read, but hang on for the good news: we can in fact make changes that keep us out of these statistics.

Studies show that studying a country's children provides the best view of that country's health. Scientists and doctors everywhere say, "This is the first generation of children not expected to outlive their parents." What? Let's read that again. "This is the first generation of children not expected to outlive their parents." It rips my heart out every time

I repeat that. My little dude is almost three, and I will do anything in my power to make sure he does not become one of these statistics because of his health. He is, however, growing up in this generation. So let us set the intention every day to teach our kids about health and detoxification and give them the tools they need to get and stay healthy.

Toxins are Cumulative

I want you to close your eyes and imagine your future children living in this environment. The odds are stacked against them. And from what we know, the main culprits are toxins. How were they even exposed to these toxins? Remember the study that evaluated the cord blood of newborns? At birth, babies carry up to three hundred chemicals in their systems, and everyday life adds to that an unbearable amount of other toxins.

> At birth, babies carry up to three hundred chemicals in their systems, and everyday life adds to that an unbearable amount of other toxins.

I have a fun analogy from Dr. Pompa that I want to share, as it helps to clarify the accumulation of toxins.

INFLAMMATION IS BIGGER THAN WE THOUGHT

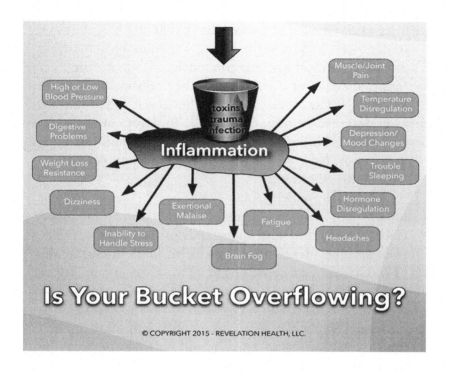

Imagine every cell in your body as a tiny little bucket. As you encounter toxins, the bucket starts filling up. You received toxins passed from your parents, including heavy metals, Perfluorooctanoic Acid chemicals or PFOAs, and more. Then, add in vaccines and possibly baby formula (with glyphosate). You ate healthy fruits and vegetables, but they were covered in pesticides. Then you went to a moldy school, followed by a moldy apartment in your twenties, four amalgam fillings from your dentist, and your bucket just kept filling, filling, filling. Finally, physical trauma or emotional stress shakes the bucket and it overflows. "Overflow" is considered when you exhibit symptoms or receive the diagnosis of a specific condition.

Symptoms don't necessarily point to a specific diagnosis. They could include simple problems such as headaches, fatigue, brain fog, exertional malaise (e.g., unusual fatigue after working out), or the inability to handle stress. Let's be honest, we always want to blame our stress on something else. "Oh, I'm just working too much," "We're moving," "A family member is sick," "It's baseball season," and so on. We all have a thousand activities, but at the end of the day, God designed us to handle stress. So if your stress levels exceed your ability to handle them, inflammation may be at the root. Now you can stop stressing about your stress and handle the cause!

Digestive problems, high or low blood pressure, joint or muscle pain, temperature abnormalities, depression, mood changes, sleep difficulty, and of course, hormone dysregulation, are all evidence of cellular inflammation. How many of you have tried to lose weight by working out and eating well and didn't drop a pound? This reflects weight loss resistance, a real condition we'll tap into later that involves hormonal imbalance. All of these are symptoms signal a bucket overflowing with toxins and inflammation leading to disease, if it hasn't already come to that.

If your body is full of toxins, inflammation will affect your future children and can possibly even hinder you from getting pregnant. Let's review a few of the most important toxins.

As you read through the rest of this section, keep in mind that solutions exist for dealing with toxins. Instead of feeling instantly overwhelmed, take heart. Not only will I teach about all of the lurking toxins, I will walk you through a healing journey so that you emerge confident and prepared to grow a healthy human—all the while getting stronger and healthier, because you deserve it too.

We will talk about food, chemicals in our water, household items, and of course give you strategies for eliminating problems in these areas. Depending on your goals and your starting point, take note of if you are a full-out, cold-turkey kind of girl or maybe you like to implement one change at a time. If you find more success accomplishing your goals one change at a time, consider designating a calendar for your health journey and map out the changes you want to implement, and when. I personally use stickers all over my calendar to keep it colorful and fun, but before you laugh, remember we have to do whatever it takes to reclaim our health, and I personally am more likely to stick to something if I can make some fun out of it!

Glyphosate

Let's first discuss glyphosate, one of the most toxic chemicals. In 1996, excitement surrounded the newly created "Roundup Ready Soybeans." Simply put, scientists genetically modified a soybean plant for resistance to Roundup (with a main chemical component of glyphosate). This enabled a farmer to spray his crops with Roundup to kill the weeds that normally would choke a crop, while the soybeans lived. While considered a breakthrough in technology, it was not without consequence. Monsanto, an international agriculture and biotechnology corporation with highly questionable integrity, launched this pseudo-plant. We now have thousands of genetically modified organisms (GMOs) or GMO products that contain glyphosate sprayed on crops. As we ingest these products, we in turn intake glyphosate into our bodies.

Glyphosate is a broad-spectrum systemic herbicide and crop desiccant (sprayed on crops such as wheat or potatoes before harvest to increase their yield). It kills weeds, especially annual broadleaf weeds and grasses that compete with crops. This occurs when it interferes with the shikimate pathway, a pathway that exists in plants and microorganisms, but not in the genome of mammals. Breathing a pesticide will irritate the nose and throat and can cause nausea and vomiting. Many detailed studies show a deeper connection between this specific pesticide and other negative health effects.

What does glyphosate do to the human body? In 2009, the *Journal of Toxicology* published research showing the mutagenic effect of glyphosate in human cell lines, while a study in 2014 explains the mechanism of damage DNA by glyphosate. It causes damage on many levels, yet its capacity upon exposure to drive mercury and aluminum deeper into cells perhaps constitutes the worst effect. Remember this as we take a deeper dive into mercury and aluminum later in the book. We know heavy metals drive brain inflammation, contribute to Types 2 and 3 diabetes, and trigger genes associated with Alzheimer's disease and dementia. They also kill bacteria needed for neurotransmitters such as serotonin and dopamine, so they mess with your gut and your brain, literally making us depressed, anxious, or afflicted with any other type of mental condition.

This graph shows that as glyphosate increased from 1989 onward, so did deaths from dementia. You can't deny this trend my friends, and many other researchers are proving, the more glyphosate used, the more people diagnosed with dementia, and premature death that it ultimately leads to. Dementia no longer only strikes people in their 70s and 80s. Doctors diagnose people as young as sixteen years of age with it.

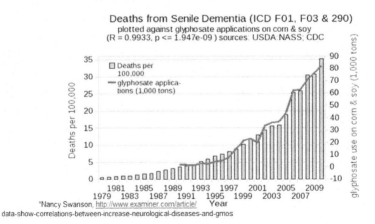

*Nancy Swanson, http://www.examiner.com/article/data-show-correlations-between-increase-neurological-diseases-and-gmos

You may wonder how our USDA and FDA would possibly allow substances like glyphosate in our food. Have you heard of the Monsanto Protection Act? Part of bill H.R.933 that Obama signed in 2013, protects large, biotech Monsanto-based companies from litigation. Prior to this bill's signature, the USDA was responsible for testing the safety of products, while the federal government still held the right to halt the testing or sale of a product suspected to jeopardize public health. In 2015, Congress passed H.R.1599, releasing companies from the obligation to label or disclose genetic engineering of their products. It also prevented any state or local law against prohibiting the growth of genetically engineered (GE) crops in their territory. Clearly the health of our future generations did not hold priority concern for anyone who helped these bills pass.

Since glyphosate is not regulated, let's talk about its presence in various foods, so you can avoid it as much as possible. According to the USDA, 90 percent of all of our soy, corn, and cotton are genetically modified and will contain glyphosate. We can safely say that anything containing these ingredients contains glyphosate. To drastically decrease your pesticide exposure, eat organic, non-GMO foods.

Look at the ingredients on everything you buy. When my son was born he was allergic/intolerant to corn. I could not even eat organic corn when I was nursing—it made his skin break out within minutes. So when I started looking for corn products in ingredients it blew my mind. It felt like everything contained either corn syrup or corn starch! How about the animals that eat chemically sprayed GMO grains and corn? Their meat now contains glyphosate.

> To drastically decrease your pesticide exposure, eat organic, non-GMO foods.

Most infant formulas contain some form of soy or soy lecithin, even if dairy forms the protein isolate as whey, we know both are loaded with glyphosate. That goes for many types of protein bars and shakes as well. Almost all wheat has been genetically modified; our environment has changed so much that the original wheat God created has been changed to survive. My favorite explanation of this is chapter 2 in *Wheat Belly*: "Not Your Grandma's Muffins: The Creation of Modern Wheat." We also know that canola oil contains glyphosate, and that is added to darn near everything. Even some potatoes and other root vegetables receive Roundup desiccation. So it also sinks into the soil and makes its way into water sources. Anyone else think this list is getting crazy long?

You can find many other resources about glyphosate and health from a brilliant researcher here: Stephanie Seneff's Home Page (mit.edu).

How do you know if you've been exposed to glyphosate? I have a really amazing resource through a company called Vibrant America. They provide an easy, mail-in urine test that checks for many toxins in addition to glyphosate. I ran this test on myself before and after detox, and then I ran the test on my two-year-old son. With my understanding of many of the toxins we have talked about, I thought I had done a pretty stellar job keeping toxins away from my kiddo. I honestly felt nervous but excited about testing him. I want to share his test with you, because I see the value in testing no matter how much you've learned about toxins. We had some work to do after his results, so I am glad I tested him. A baseline helps; remember knowledge is power. Tests simply give us information to move forward. They are not a diagnosis or a sentence.

Environmental Toxins Summary

Environmental Toxins - High

Test Name	In Control	Moderate	High	Current Level	Previous Level
Dimethylphosphate (DMP) (mcg/g)	≤5.20	5.21-37.19	≥37.20	95.36	
mono-(2-ethyl-5-hydroxyhexyl) phthalate (MEHHP) (mcg/g)	≤42.00	42.01-168.99	≥169.00	573.88	
Bisphenol A (BPA) (mcg/g)	≤3.20	3.21-10.80	≥10.81	27.16	

Environmental Toxins - Moderate

Test Name	In Control	Moderate	High	Current Level	Previous Level
Glyphosate (mcg/g)	≤0.75	0.76-2.29	≥2.30	1.36	
3-Phenoxybenzoic Acid (3PBA) (mcg/g)	≤0.57	0.58-6.39	≥6.40	3.28	
Tiglylglycine (TG) (mcg/g)	≤0.10	0.11-11.29	≥11.30	5.68	
2-Hydroxyisobutyric Acid (2HIB) (mcg/g)	≤1005.00	1005.01-5789.99	≥5790.00	4566.15	

Check out some of these other toxins that my poor little two-year-old has been exposed to. We will talk in detail about some of the other ones in the Avoiding Plastics section in Chapter 6.

I would like to highlight another result: Dimethylphosphate (DMP), a pesticide found even on some organic fruits and vegetables. Since pesticides kill bugs, why would they not affect humans, especially when we find their residues found in almost all of the food we consume? Many studies research pesticides and their contribution to our children's declining health. However, I want to highlight one that thoroughly studies the direct correlation of pesticide exposure and ADHD. This study in Denmark tested the pesticide levels of 948 pregnant women, then followed their children until two to four years of age. They found that mothers with higher levels of pesticides had much higher chances of their children expressing ADHD symptoms. While the mechanism still needs study, these researchers speculated that pesticides may simply turn on a genetic propensity for ADHD. Ahh, does this all begin to fit together? Refer back to the study about mice and their DNA if you have forgotten.

We know that hundreds of chemicals every year are banned from organic use, but simply buying organic is not good enough. You need to wash your fruits, veggies, and your bread. (Ha! Just kidding on the bread comment. I wanted to make sure you were still paying attention.) Since you can't wash bread, use the non-GMO, organic label to avoid as many hormone-disrupting, cancer-causing, brain-fogging chemicals as possible.

Fluoride

Toothpaste companies advertise fluoride in toothpaste as some believe that it improves our teeth. It turns out, though, that fluoride is a hazardous by-product of fertilizer.

Fluoride is linked to the following conditions:

- Lower IQ in children
- Learning disabilities
- Behavioral disorders
- Rapid aging
- Decrease in bone density and strength
- Metabolic dysfunction
- Autoimmune disease
- Cognitive decline
- Increased risk of cancer

Fluoride poses a significant danger due to its effect on thyroid function. Whenever I search for the truth of a doctor or scientist's statement, I look for it to include information on a mechanism of action. So let's get down to the biochemistry. *The Case Against Fluoride* by Paul Connett provides excellent resources with evidence that fluoride interferes with thyroid function. I encourage you to read the book, as I list and summarize only a few points here.

1. **Fluoride-induced goiter.** Fluoride mimics iodine and boots it out of its rightful position on the T3 and T4 hormones, leading to malfunction and swelling of the thyroid gland.

2. **Treatment of hyperthyroid patents.** Between 1920–1950, doctors used fluoride to suppress an overactive thyroid. So what happens if people have normal thyroid function? It gets suppressed, and you create an epidemic of people with *hypo*thyroid conditions.

3. **Low iodide and brain development.**
More fluoride = low iodide = higher possibility of developmental disabilities in children whose mothers ingest fluoride during pregnancy.

4. **Thyroid stimulating hormone (TSH).** Basically, fluoride can mimic and therefore displace TSH, the hormone secreted by your brain that gives your thyroid instructions, in certain situations.

Since the thyroid factors significantly into a healthy pregnancy, healthy babies, and a healthy postpartum period; it is vital to know the sources of fluoride and limit your exposure as much as possible.

Sources of Fluoride

1. Fluoridated water supplies.
2. Toothpaste enhanced with fluoride. Check the label of your toothpaste: Does it have a caution or even a poison label on it? Children have literally died because they ate a whole tube of toothpaste.
3. Mouthwash enhanced with fluoride.
4. Fluoride supplements. Oh yes, I took the tiny purple pills our pediatrician recommended as a child.
5. Food processed with fluoridated water. Whatever water you use in cooking transmits its chemicals into your food.

So how did we get this so wrong? In the late 1960s, Florida passed emission laws because fluorine from the phosphate industry was causing harm to citrus trees and creating fluorosis in cattle (severe problems with the cow's dental and skeletal systems). They came up with ways to decrease it in the air, but then had tankers full of fluoride, a product they then *sold* for "water fluoridation." It is estimated that 90% of water systems in the US are fluoridated. Super long story short, the researchers argued over its effectiveness in strengthening teeth, its need for oral ingestion vs. topical application, then that its presence in toothpaste would negate its need in our water supply. This battle still continues with the truth hidden in many prominent sources of information. Page 261 quotes Michael Connett as he interviews Dr. William Hirzy. He speaks to the notion that the truth remains hidden because the big players of the

> CDC, the ADA, and other large organizations profit from their "fear of losing credibility" argument for continuing public exposure to fluoride. He states that "Putting this stuff in the drinking water is in essence just a hazardous waste management tool. It has nothing to do with dental health whatsoever. It has to do with defending the reputation of people who have been promoting fluoridation for years and years and years and now find themselves way out on a limb and have nothing more to say except 'safe and effective,' 'safe and effective,' 'safe and effective,' when in fact it is neither safe nor effective. But they can't change. They are riding a tiger and can't get off."

Lead

Lead is a naturally occurring metal found in the earth, but not intended to land inside our bodies. It has been used in paint, gasoline, plumbing pipes, batteries, cosmetics, and many other unexpected places. It acts as a potent neurotoxin known to contribute to decreased learning, shortened attention span, memory challenges, irritability, fatigue, and as exposure increases, it can lead to severe neurological complications or death. According to a 2020 report by the United Nations Children's Fund (UNICEF), lead causes over 900,000 premature deaths in adults every year.

In 2013, the World Health Organization (WHO) stated, "Lead is a cumulative toxicant that affects multiple body systems and is particularly harmful to young children. There is no level of exposure to lead that is known to be without harmful effects." By referring to lead as a "cumulative toxicant," they acknowledge that it builds in our bodies with exposure. Because the body's job is survival, it takes lead out of our blood and stores it in deeper tissues, like our bones and brain.

Perhaps the sneakiest form of lead exposure occurs in utero from mom to baby. Heavy metals pass down for four generations. Thank you, Mom, Dad, Grandma, Grandpa, other Grandma, and other Grandpa. And thank you to four sets of great-grandparents for passing these toxins on. They're accumulating. Lead turns on bad genes associated with many diseases and even obesity for four generations. Since it's stored in our bones, lead leaches out of bone into our other tissues when we move through hormonal changes like puberty, pregnancy, and menopause when bone density is lost or remodeling. So, as you grow a tiny human, whatever metals or other toxins you have in your body leach out and enter your baby.

> **Heavy metals pass down for four generations.**

These images show the provoked-urine challenge results from a mother and a son. The son was 5 years old, never vaccinated, drank clean water, lived with lead-free toys and paints, and the parents carefully monitored their environment. All that to say that even though the child had limited exposure once out of the womb, he still inherited half of his mother's lead.

MOTHER

Metal	Result	Reference Range	Result	Reference Range	Chart
Arsenic	21	< 130	31	< 140	
Beryllium	< dl	< 0.5	< dl	< 0.6	
Bismuth	< dl	< 15	< dl	< 15	
Cadmium	0.4	< 2	0.6	< 2	
Lead	47	< 5	69	< 5	
Mercury	1.3	< 4	1.9	< 5	
Nickel	8.3	< 12	12	< 15	
Platinum	< dl	< 1	< dl	< 1	
Thallium	0.1	< 0.8	0.1	< 0.7	
Thorium	< dl	< 0.3	< dl	< 0.3	
Tin	1.7	< 10	2.4	< 9	
Tungsten	< dl	< 1	< dl	< 0.9	
Uranium	< dl	< 0.2	< dl	< 0.2	

	RESULT mg/24 hr	REFERENCE RANGE	2SD LOW	1SD LOW	MEAN	1SD HIGH	2SD HIGH

SON

POTENTIALLY TOXIC METALS

METALS	RESULT µg/g CREAT	REFERENCE RANGE	WITHIN REFERENCE RANGE	ELEVATED	VERY ELEVATED
Aluminum	< dl	< 60			
Antimony	0.3	< 1.5			
Arsenic	34	< 130			
Beryllium	< dl	< 0.6			
Bismuth	< dl	< 20			
Cadmium	0.5	< 2			
Lead	32	< 5			
Mercury	1.7	< 5			
Nickel	17	< 15			
Platinum	< dl	< 1			
Thallium	< dl	< 1.1			
Thorium	< dl	< 0.5			
Tin	1	< 15			
Tungsten	1.3	< 1.5			
Uranium	< dl	< 0.2			

In 2016, China produced an excellent study of close to 4,000 people, specifically evaluating the negative effects of lead on the sex hormones of men and women. They concluded that lead crosses the blood–brain barrier and directly affects the hypothalamic–pituitary function, which plays an important role in regulating sex hormones. The second mechanism in play consists of the indirect effect of homocysteine levels on sex hormones; interestingly, women with PCOS also have elevated levels of homocysteine and definitely do not have balanced sex hormones. We understand, then, that lead factors substantially into infertility. I believe we need to promote awareness of the dangers of heavy metals in the reproductive world.

Time Magazine ran an article entitled "The Poisoning of an American City." You may remember the tragic stories of Flint, Michigan, where children died from high lead levels in their water. Here's the crazy thing, even though we only heard about Flint, they weren't alone. Ninety-eight public water systems in California reported high levels of lead between 2012 and 2000. Eighteen cities in Pennsylvania, including Pittsburgh, had higher lead levels than Flint. Lead resides in old pipes, and fluoride in the water supply leaches lead from the pipes, pulling it into your water. In chapter 6, I provide a list of resources for clean water.

Let's talk about some simpler means of lead exposure. Did you know that most lipsticks contain lead? The FDA posted a chart with lipsticks, by brand, listing the lead amounts each contained as a part of a 2007 study.

FDA Analyses of Lead in Lipsticks – Initial Survey

The following results for lead content in a selection of lipsticks were obtained by scientists at the U.S. Food and Drug Administration (FDA) and reported in the *Journal of Cosmetic Science* disclaimer icon. FDA purchased lipsticks from retail stores between October and December 2007.

Sample #	Brand	Parent company	Lipstick line Shade # Shade[a]	Lot #[b]	Lead (Pb)[c] (ppm)[d]
1a	Cover Girl	Procter & Gamble	Incredifull Lipcolor 964 Maximum Red	7241S1	3.06
1b	Cover Girl	Procter & Gamble	Incredifull Lipcolor 964 Maximum Red	5188S1	3.05
	Revlon	Revlon	ColorStay Lipcolor 345	Composite[e]	2.91[f]
2			Red Velvet	07298	2.38
3	Cover Girl	Procter & Gamble	Queen Collection Q580 Ruby Remix	7136	2.24

Kohl, Kahal, Surma, Tiro, Tozali, or Kwalli are eyeliner brands (popular in many parts of the world) that have an extremely high content of lead. The US prohibits their sale here, but specialty markets still sell them. Know your sources.

Did you know that most lipsticks contain lead?

The federal government (fda.gov) has more information on the regulation of these products, if regulated at all. In 1980, lead acetate was listed as a color additive for "safe" use in hair-coloring products. Not until 2018 did the FDA remove it from the safe list. Remember to run your products through EWG's Skin Deep Database. I also found an excellent article at https://ireadlabelsforyou.com/depths-skin-deep-database-cosmetics/ that discusses the limitations of the EWG and how you can optimize choices that align with the goal of growing a healthy human.

Mercury

A 2017 study published in the Environmental Research and Public Health Journal stated that even low concentrations of mercury with chronic exposure can cause cardiovascular, reproductive, and developmental toxicity; neurotoxicity; nephrotoxicity, immunotoxicity; and carcinogenicity.

Do you have silver fillings in your teeth? Did your mother have silver fillings in her teeth? Have you ever had a vaccination? A flu shot? Did you use contact solution in the 1980s? All of these contain mercury. People usually think of fish first, but fish contain a different form of mercury at much lower concentration levels than the substances mentioned above.

Mercury is a naturally occurring element and found in three forms:

1. Metallic mercury found in thermometers, fluorescent bulbs, and amalgam fillings.
2. Inorganic mercury compounds found in beauty products and batteries.
3. Organic mercury as methylmercury found in fish, and ethylmercury in vaccines.

You may know that it was not good to play with the amazing "liquid silver" in your grandmother's thermometer, and maybe you had to clear the room after a fluorescent bulb broke at school. It is crazy to think that dentists put this same form of mercury in our teeth. Also take note of beauty products. Even if you may have minimal exposure from these, it's all about our little buckets filling and filling.

You probably know to avoid raw fish when you are pregnant or trying to get pregnant, but parasites are not the only concern. Fish can contain mercury, but instead of avoiding it altogether (we know it has beneficial nutrients), choose smaller fish, as they have lower concentrations of mercury, and also know the source of the fish. The Environmental Protection Agency EPA has a database where you can look up the source of the fish and if there are any health advisories on the toxins in that area.

Vaccines and dental vapors from amalgam fillings make the most substantial contribution to mercury overload in the human body. Go to your local dentist's office and ask to see the container that the amalgam fillings come in. It warns of neurotoxic, nephrotic effects, which means it affects your kidneys and your nervous system. It says, "Poison: corrosive—personal protection must be used. Keep out of reach of children." And guess where the dentist plans to place it? That's right—in your mouth, pretty darn close to your brain. Amalgam fillings are standard dental care, and many dentists still think that no harm comes from putting them in our mouths.

Dental amalgams consist of about 50 percent metallic mercury. Here's another scary thing: we pass it on to our babies in the womb. The European Journal of Pediatrics published a study of autopsied babies, and researchers found that the amount of mercury in the babies' brains correlated to the number of fillings in the mother's mouths. They concluded that the more amalgam fillings present in your mouth, the more mercury you'll have in your organs, including the brain, kidneys, heart, and liver. In 2005, a study of Brazilian women found that the amount of mercury in breastmilk of lactating woman correlated with the amount of amalgam fillings in the mother's mouth. There is no question that we pass this toxic metal to our children.

By the time you experience a symptom, you have probably had a problem brewing for years.

In 1988, the Environmental Protection Agency (EPA) declared scrapped dental amalgam materials as hazardous waste. The Occupation Safety and Health Administration (OSHA) mandates certain protocols for dentists handling amalgam fillings before entering and after exiting your mouth. Scrap amalgam must be stored in an unbreakable, tightly sealed container away from heat. Dentists and their assistants must follow a "no-touch" technique while handling it and must store it in liquid (preferably a glycerin-photographic-fixer solution). It is extremely toxic. On July 1, 2018, the European Union banned its use for children under fifteen as well as pregnant or nursing women. It also required each of the twenty-eight countries to submit a plan for reducing amalgam use in the remainder of the population. Whereas in America, most dentists tell you that amalgams are not toxic. They're not a problem. No, you shouldn't get your silver fillings out. That will cause you more exposure.

Take a look at this list of symptoms, and keep in mind that by the time you experience a symptom, you have probably had a problem brewing for years. In some cases, people can experience these symptoms directly after a filling, or if a filling is removed or replaced improperly, or it may take years.

Symptoms of Mercury Toxicity

- depression
- fatigue
- anxiety
- forgetfulness
- eyelid, face, or muscle twitching
- digestive issues

- constipation or diarrhea
- frequent bad breath
- constant body odor
- dizziness
- irritability
- sensitivity to sound
- inability to concentrate
- brain fog
- abnormal menses
- low body temperature
- cold hands and feet
- tender teeth
- tinnitus or ringing in the ears
- insomnia
- metallic taste in the mouth
- nail fungus
- unexplained anger
- autoimmune response

Jane came into my office, looking for help with her neck pain. We walked her through a corrective process until she graduated to maintenance care. We saw her on a fairly regular basis. Then I didn't see her for almost a year. Her husband came in to get adjusted, so I asked about Jane. He hung his head, and said, "Honestly, we're about to lose our house. Jane has developed severe anxiety over the last year. She cannot drive and struggles with daily tasks." An attorney, she was even unable to work, and they had two young daughters at home. He said it felt like their whole life was crumbling because of her debilitating anxiety.

I reached out and was so glad that Jane wanted to go through our detox process. Every month she felt better on many levels, but the anxiety persisted. Something else was at the root. I sent Jane to our biological dentist, who uses all the necessary precautions to remove amalgam fillings properly. He removed six large amalgams, and within three weeks her brain fog began to lift and the anxiety began to subside. With the source removed, we dove into a deeper detox. I'm excited to tell you that after a few rounds of detox, her anxiety disappeared, and she was able to return to work. They kept their house, and most importantly, the girls got their mama back.

No amount of CBD oil or supplementation would fix Jane's anxiety. Pharmaceuticals made her feel unlike herself, and she hated taking them. Jane's journey included detoxification, but also properly removing her amalgam fillings.

This may or may not be a part of your prep journey, but the dentist you choose is extremely important as there are many other toxins we can be exposed to at the dentist. Chapter 6 will have more details about clean dentistry.

Mercury and Our Hormones

Mercury in the human body primarily settles in the pituitary gland and hypothalamus of the brain. These control/influence the thyroid and adrenal glands. Both organs need to be in top shape to grow a human. Adrenals play a large part in regulating the sex hormones through all the hormonal changes in life including puberty, pregnancy, the postpartum phase, menopause, and beyond. If your thyroid and adrenal glands are stressed, your body will find it difficult to navigate these changes, which may show up as fatigue, anxiety, low libido, infertility, and any other symptom of your body's inability to maintain homeostasis. And if your brain is full of mercury, you can support your thyroid and adrenals until the cows come home, but this will not fix your problem.

Many fertility clinics now test for heavy metal toxicity, but sadly they do not always use proper testing, and most of them do not use safe, appropriate binders. Blood, hair, or non-provoked urine tests do not reveal what your body is genuinely storing. Results are also affected by how your eliminating pathways are working. Properly assessing heavy metals requires a provoked urine challenge. Provoked means that you take a binding agent before you collect your urine sample over 6–24 hours, to pull the metals from deeper tissues and provide a more accurate result.

If you or someone you love has struggled with infertility, endometriosis, PCOS, fibroids, or any other unresolved hormonal condition, mercury and other heavy metals could be the root cause of the

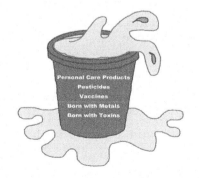

dysfunction. If you do not have any of these concerns, but you have silver fillings, I recommend their removal by a biological dentist. Then, along with those who have been vaccinated or suspect heavy metal toxicity from another source, complete the True Cellular Detox program to clean the source from your system.

Heavy Metals in "Shots"

The amount of aluminum the FDA considers medically "safe" in an infant IV drip is 30 micrograms over a 24-hour period. Yet one hepatitis B vaccine contains 250 micrograms, given within twelve hours of birth. By two months of age, infants get five to eight more shots, totaling 1,200 to 2,000 micrograms of aluminum. But wait! You said FDA considers only 30 micrograms as safe. This constitutes a serious problem, and only you as the parent can do something about it.

Vaccines contain aluminum because it can cross the blood–brain barrier and take the virus or other component of vaccines into deeper tissues. All vaccines contain some kind of "driver" or adjuvant intended to make the vaccine more effective in evoking antibodies. Preservatives such as thimerosal or mercury improve the shelf life of vaccines, yet we just discussed the devastating cumulative effects of these substances to our brain and body. Dr. Hugh Fudenburg was "one of the world's leading immunologists and the thirteenth most quoted biologist of our time, appearing in nearly 850 papers in peer-reviewed journals." This man knew his stuff! He stated that "if an individual had five consecutive flu shots between 1970 and 1980, they had a ten times greater chance of developing Alzheimer's disease." When asked why, he replied that "gradually mercury and aluminum build up in the brain," and then you pass it on. The first sign is short term memory loss and brain fog, now called pre-dementia. Dementia and Alzheimer's disease are the fastest growing diseases in the United States and the third cause of death. While you may not be thinking now of diseases that typically occur later in life, understanding how they develop gives us power for intentional prevention. I know some employers require flu shots, but in my opinion, you should do anything you can to avoid them.

In 1986, The National Childhood Vaccine Injury Act bill passed, absolving all vaccine manufacturers from responsibility of persons who experience injury or death from a vaccine. Basically, you can't sue them if you or your child is injured. With no accountability, manufacturers have added hundreds of additives to vaccines that harm our children. Even pediatricians and other doctors are not aware of all vaccine ingredients and the implications for your health. Only the doctors researching and investigating the ingredients will understand the consequences. If you have concern over your child's vaccine schedule, check with your state's laws. I believe forty-six states still have a religious and a philosophical exemption allowing your child to attend school or any other public place no matter your decision on vaccines. You don't even need a doctor's note—just your parental signature. Remember, you hold the right as a parent to do what is best for your child. I also believe it is important for a parent to feel respected and supported as they make these important decisions for their families. I encourage people to keep searching until they find both in a physician.

Vaccines don't just cause issues with children. When you get pregnant, if you decide to see an obstetrician, they will most likely recommend a flu shot (depending on the time of year), and a Tdap vaccine for tetanus, diphtheria, and pertussis. The CDC recommends one shot for every

> Understanding how diseases like dementia and Alzheimer's develop gives us power for intentional prevention.

pregnancy, claiming it will protect the baby through the mother. This theory presents many problems, including the unknown effects to a woman and her baby after multiple Tdaps, along with the accumulation of metals. I encourage you to research the ingredients of this vaccine before consenting. It specifically contains aluminum, formaldehyde, and many other DNA-damaging components you do not want surrounding your child in the womb. When you research vaccines and see an ingredient such as HEK-293 or MRC-5, or any other combination of letters and numbers, conduct an internet search and study them. They will not directly list aborted fetal or embryonic tissue or many other controversial additives in the ingredients—they will code them.

Dr. Sherry Tenpenny, a medical doctor with a very impressive background, offers an excellent online course for vaccines during pregnancy at vaccineu.com. She provides access to thousands of research articles regarding health and vaccines. Take a few of her courses, then pass them on to any family member who questions your decisions! I personally took the pregnancy series and the RhoGAM module when I was pregnant, and I was extremely impressed.

It might feel funny now to joke about the forgetfulness of your kids or your husband, but now knowing that metals drive brain inflammation and ultimately affect brain function, it may make you think. We cannot ignore the serious culprit of heavy metals and brain fog, and it is nothing short of tragic, that we can't trust organizations established to protect people. We have to take responsibility for our own health, and do our own research!

Food Intolerance and Allergies

Let's say researchers want to study food allergies in rats. If they want to provoke a peanut allergy in the rat, they administer an injection with a peanut protein and aluminum. Because aluminum drives the protein into the body crossing barriers at a cellular level, the body will create an autoimmune reaction, or allergy, to that substance. If your child's vaccine contains aluminum (nearly all do), along with egg proteins, dairy proteins, and many other ingredients you would never give your infant, it will create allergies to those substances in your child. Then, they also don't tell you that the aluminum-filled vaccine will drive whatever your child has eaten (a peanut butter and jelly sandwich, or chicken and avocado, etc.) through gut membranes they're not supposed to cross, and *voilà*, they become allergic or intolerant to all those foods. If you suffer with food allergies or perhaps have a child with sensitivities, you know firsthand how they can run your life. You can't eat anywhere, and the minute you eat at a friend's house out of politeness, you find yourself running to the bathroom, or sick the entire next day because your body can't handle normal foods.

We know that food allergies or food intolerances lead to autoimmune conditions. Autoimmunity occurs when your immune system attacks your own body. If your immune system is weak, you are in deep trouble. We always feel we should just push through, that it is just temporary. I recommend getting to the cause of the immune dysfunction—it's a beautiful thing when you detoxify metals properly and the immune system comes back online!

Mold

Maybe this sounds like you or someone you know: it didn't use to feel so difficult to accomplish simple tasks, so unbearable to make it through a day at work, and now you find it impossible to finish a load of laundry, you're so tired all the time. Maybe you've been to countless doctors and had countless tests, only to be told that everything is normal, or that you just have allergies, or maybe even worse . . . you look fine, so your complaints and symptoms must be in your head. Countless people with digestive disorders have searched for answers, only to be told, "There is nothing wrong with your stomach. You're just depressed" or "You have a psychological problem," aka "It's all in your head." Too many people have experienced this disrespect and not had their real condition addressed. Very often we find mold toxicity when a condition seems inexplicable.

Mold is a biotoxin and creates inflammation in your nervous system, and since your nervous system controls everything in your body, it affects every system, and the symptoms don't always fit into an easy diagnosis. Mold is a fungus that begins as tiny spores. When an environment supports its growth, it multiplies. Mold is found in basements, crawlspaces, basically anywhere water can reach, including the space in between walls, behind cupboards or under sinks. Sometimes you notice a musty smell, and at other times the smell is undetectable even with mold present. Some people with greater mold sensitivity seem to have a higher toxic load and/or challenged immune system. Mold made the top three list of primary culprits causing illness, along with heavy metals and hidden infections. These three serve as the true root causes of almost every inflammatory condition.

If you want to check your home for mold effectively, consider ordering an Environmental Relative Moldiness

Index (ERMI) test. If you know that your childhood home, school, or workplace had mold; it remains in your system and could still affect your health today. I consulted with a young lady diagnosed with Hashimoto's disease at eleven years of age. She was struggling with her energy levels at age sixteen. She went on to explain that she felt the worst on days that she had to travel for golf. She said after the trip to a match, she would want nothing more than to lie down and take a nap. Her mother found out that the van transporting the athletes had water damage and was full of mold. Keeping her out of the van has helped her energy tremendously. However, we now need to work on detoxing her body on a deeper level.

> When we keep asking the right questions, we find the root cause.

I believe the most important thing to learn when navigating your health is ask why: "Okay, so my thyroid numbers are not normal, why is that?" Is your thyroid under-functioning, or is your liver unable to convert T4 to the active T3? Maybe your HPA axis isn't working well and it's more of a brain inflammation issue. When we keep asking the right questions, we find the root cause. We discover hidden problems such as metals in the deeper tissues, mold, and infections (e.g., Lyme, root canals, cavitations from tooth extraction, and so on). Then, if you have the right practitioner, you can plug in and play the right strategies to regain your health.

CHAPTER 3
WHAT ARE TOXINS REALLY AFFECTING?

Toxins, toxins, toxins. Are you sick of that word yet? This has become an overwhelming topic, but we can't ignore it since inflammation caused by toxins lies at the true root of all disease and dysfunction. When you intentionally researching toxins before growing your humans, you have a unique opportunity to set them up for the healthiest life possible. We, in fact, live in the most toxic generation known to mankind, and our kids suffer as they develop disease at record low ages.

Oxford Dictionary defines a toxin as "an antigenic poison or venom of plant or animal origin, especially one produced or derived from microorganisms and causing disease when present at low concentrations in the body." When you are thinking about growing humans, you must understand that you are their environment.

You — Your Baby's Environment

Thousands of chemicals and toxins affect your health, and just as one hundred different medications could have one hundred different mechanisms of action and one hundred different side effects, so can toxins. Some pass through our bodily fluids, while some wreak havoc on our DNA as they leave our bodies. Some stay for months or years, and some, like heavy metals, will find a home in our deeper tissues like the gut, bone, and brain.

When I began this journey, I googled "what to do before getting pregnant." I found an article written by an obstetrician who listed ten things to do before getting pregnant and contained typical information like stop taking birth control, and stop smoking, but it also encouraged the removal of toxins from your environment. I thought, *Wow, it's about time they are talking about this!* The article went on to discuss the toxicity of vitamin A found in many beauty products. Another source similarly warned against the toxicity of too much vitamin D. Very few of the articles even mentioned pesticides or other endocrine-disrupting chemicals, which of course added fuel to my fire to get this information to you.

We know that vitamins A, D, E, and K are fat-soluble vitamins, and it was assumed for quite some time that you could overdose on these vitamins. But we also know that our food is deficient in nutrients, our bodies are deficient, and the more toxic we are, the more deficient we become. It's highly unlikely that one would consume toxic levels of these essential vitamins unless it was an unusual situation. In my opinion, these articles should explore the toxins in our air, our water, our food, our clothing, and our cleaning supplies, as these are the real offenders that affect our ability to conceive and damage the DNA of our future children.

The other nine items addressed in this article, in my opinion did not present enough detail, and for someone who eats well, doesn't smoke, and doesn't take birth control pills, it provided little useful information. After this, I sat down and mapped out everything I planned to do before growing my next human.

In the chapters ahead, we will address toxins that directly affect your hormones. It's important to recognize that many other countries have banned hundreds of chemicals that we still use in the United States. I'm talking about commonly used items such as toothpaste and shampoo. Toxins cause perhaps the most detrimental changes to our DNA. We now have brilliant research showing that specific toxins can alter genetic expression. And we know that toxins can turn on bad genes and turn off good ones, therefore setting your body on a pathway to disease.

Epigenetic Studies on DNA

Think for a minute of the laundry list of health conditions in your family. In mine alone, we have kidney disease, heart disease, multiple types of cancer, thyroid issues, obesity, and the list goes on and on. I'm sure yours does too. Medicine has conditioned us to think that your family history determines your health outcome. Rather than looking for causes, too many people search for a quick fix. Some women, for example, will opt for a mastectomy just because their mother and grandmother had breast cancer. They see it as a way to prevent cancer in the future. Instead of electing to have an extreme procedure, I prefer to look for the causes of the cancer and work from that angle.

In 2019, researchers at Duke University exposed mice to a toxin similar to glyphosate. It turned on a specific gene, causing the mice to become morbidly obese and develop thyroid conditions as well as heart disease. Researchers repeated the study on twin mice. All the mice followed the same diet and exercise regimen, but only one set of twins received exposure to the toxin. The result? The group exposed to the toxin became morbidly obese and developed thyroid conditions as well as heart disease. The mice in the research study reproduced, and the healthy mice gave birth to healthy babies. The sick mice gave birth to sick babies. By removing the toxin from the mice's environment and repairing their DNA, however, researchers enabled the mice to recover their health. They lost weight, their hair changed color (a positive marker), and their thyroid conditions and heart disease improved. When these mice reproduced, they had healthy babies.

This is extremely important because it provides me with hope that the ball is in our court. Skyrocketing disease statistics and a family history peppered with a long list of diseases and medical conditions ultimately don't matter. We *can* act to change our DNA. I might have the kidney disease gene, the hyperthyroid gene, the heart disease gene—any or all of these—but that doesn't guarantee their activation. You may have had no idea how your daily choices affect your DNA (another reason I'm so passionate about this), because the controlling effect of toxins on health blindsides so many. No matter how many organic vegetables you put in your body, if you expose yourself to toxins, you set yourself on a course for disease.

> **Skyrocketing disease statistics and a family history peppered with a long list of diseases and medical conditions ultimately don't matter. *We can act to change our DNA.***

God made our bodies to constantly remove waste and toxins. We have amazing organs and systems that solely work to filter and eliminate toxins—the liver, kidneys, lymph nodes, and perhaps the most famous one, our gut. All of these parts work together to eliminate the toxins we encounter. The problem comes when our bodies cannot handle the sheer load of toxins we have, or determine how to eliminate foreign toxins. When either of these happen, our body stores the toxins in the deepest tissues, such as bone, to protect itself. The body's main job, after all, is survival.

Imagine having almost three hundred chemicals inside your body before you ever take your first breath. No wonder our organs get bogged down. And over time, stronger chemical and toxin exposure means deeper tissue storage. The subject of toxins can produce great frustration, especially when we feel deceived and blindsided by so many companies, agencies, institutions, and habits we trust in, or take for granted. Many large companies—even those with household names or that profess themselves as green or environmentally friendly—have a surprising amount of ingredients toxic to the human body. There is, however, a light on the end of the tunnel, and the process of detoxing does not have to be overwhelming. It becomes a journey.

I truly believe that when we empower ourselves with the truth and get on mission to grow a healthy family, teaching our children a vibrant lifestyle, we will rise above and be the exceptions to society's downward trend in disease. As we will discuss in later chapters, appropriate testing and detoxification will significantly help, but removing the source of the toxin is paramount. Let's break this down.

The 5 Rs of Cellular Healing

Dr. Dan Pompa teaches the 5 Rs, or principles, of detoxification across the country. This is a beautiful method of breaking down the detoxification process at a cellular level. You can find the nuts and bolts of his teaching at his website, drpompa.com. After the Flint, Michigan, crisis, he taught doctors there how to properly detox the children from lead. His own story of failing health and recovery drives him to teach other practitioners. He and his partners created a platform where they can learn from the brightest minds, collaborate, and obtain real answers to patient concerns (visit Health Centers of the Future at HCFseminars.com). Several levels of learning from seminars to detox certifications, to deeper functional training exist; I am proud to participate in the Platinum Elite group of doctors that Dr. Pompa pours into weekly. You would greatly benefit from checking out his YouTube channel and *Cellular Healing TV* podcast. He finds the greatest minds in the world and interviews them so you can learn the most cutting-edge strategies for healing yourself and your family. Here I break down his 5Rs, critical to restoring your health.

R1: Remove the Source

This might sound like a no brainer, and maybe your first thought is, "Okay, I should probably stop cleaning with Clorox bleach," but toxins we find in more than just cleaning products. Self-care products, cosmetics, soaps, and toothpastes all contain toxins. External sources like silver fillings, teeth sealants, vaccinations, and flu shots as well as toxic chemicals and molds found in the environment also produce toxins. We can clean many of these sources up without testing. But if you are ready to identify the main culprits in your toxic load, let's address some of the most accurate and productive ways to test for toxins.

You can easily test environmental toxins. Check Section 2 in the "Glyphosate" chapter for a picture of my son's test. Again the company Vibrant America offers a urine test that requires you to collect a sample and send it in for analysis. They return a very detailed report, covering multiple sources of BPAs, phthalates, pesticides, glyphosate, and many other toxins found in everyday life. With it, you can uncover some of your most important triggers.

Vibrant America also offers an amazing mycotoxin test covering biotoxins (to see if you have had mold exposure, and if so, what kind). A provoked-urine challenge most accurately evaluates heavy metals in the body, and they offer this test as well (as does Doctor's Data). *Provoked-urine challenge* means that a patient takes a binding supplement that pulls metals into the urine for testing. You will most likely need a practitioner to order this test so they can set the proper dose of the provoking agent. Because deeper tissues store heavy metals, looking for them in blood, hair, or urine without a provoking agent will not provide an accurate measurement of your levels. Each of these tests gives you better insight, which allows you to embark upon a more detailed detox program.

If testing is not an immediate option, I suggest you first download an app. Yes, there is an app for that. "Think Dirty" allows you to scan products, which receive a score of one to ten (ten being the most toxic). You really don't want to use anything greater than a four on your body—especially when it comes to things you put on your body, clothes, or dishes. After you download this app, go into your bathroom and start scanning products. Make two piles, one for health-promoting items, and another for toxic products. I would encourage you to throw away everything toxic and start from scratch if you have to. No matter what you've invested in a product, it is not worth your health. This is probably when the little voice of doubt will creep in and say, "Oh, those things aren't really that bad, right?" My best answer is yes. Some products can be *that bad*.

> **No matter what you've invested in a product, it is not worth your health.**

As you start the detoxing process, view it as a valuable opportunity. This is your chance to set new priorities and teach your children and other loved ones what they should put on and in their bodies, and what they should not.

One group of chemicals used in many personal care products are parabens. Ten years ago, I did not know that they potentially stay in your body for life. Parabens serve as a preservative, widely used in many types of cosmetics, lotions, shampoos, and other toiletries. They cause problems because they mimic estrogen in our bodies, particularly when they drive estrogen dominant cancers. Doctors have extracted tumors from women's breasts and literally found intact parabens inside the tumor. *What?* That means that, components of the lovely, popular mall-brand body lotion that you used religiously every day of high school are actually still with you. Those parabens are still intact in your tissues, even though you just applied them to your skin. Many countries have banned these same parabens for children and pregnant women. Because I am keenly aware that parabens, sulfates, BPA, and phthalates are found in multiple baby products, I also tested my son after I saw my report. At two-and-a-half years of age, he fell on the moderate-to-high scale for many of these toxins. Those results tell us that he could have been born with some of them, from me, or that his tiny body was exposed to these toxins after birth, and they're already wreaking havoc at a cellular level. Every single day. Getting a report like this for your child or even yourself can overwhelm you, but for me, I feared not knowing much more than knowing. I had to know to make better choices for my son. Knowledge is power, and in this case, knowledge could mean a path of health or a path of disease.

We will naturally excrete some toxins through stool, urine, sweat, and blood. Many will stay in our body until we have a specific, intentional detoxification with products that cross gut barriers and blood–brain barriers, effectively binding to and eliminating the toxins. Herbal cleanses and supplements can help in some situations, but in some people, they can actually make symptoms worse.

R2: Regenerate the Cell Membrane

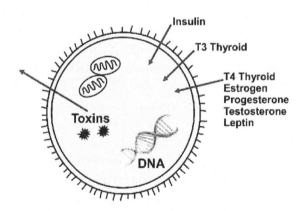

A phospholipid bilayer, essentially fat, makes up our cell membranes. Remember, fats store toxins. As cell membranes become inflamed, their receptors for all of your hormones become blocked. Repairing this membrane means decreasing bad fats and increasing good ones. The ratio of good to bad fats needs to be at least 70 to 30 percent, just to fight off oxidative damage and cancer, but you should ideally aim for 80 percent good fats.

Repairing the membrane requires supplementation, which can mean an actual supplement or pill, but the best strategy involves adding good fats to your everyday diet. Try some of these:

- Saturated fats and cholesterol—yes those egg yolks are good for you
- Ghee

- Grass-fed and grass-finished beef
- Organic olive oils
- Avocado or almond oil for use with higher heat
- Coconut oil

Brian Peskin, a brilliant professor whom I interviewed, wrote a book explaining essential oils and non-essential oils. In short, according to Peskin, if you take fish oil, you are consuming bad fats, creating inflammation, and even increasing the chances of cancerous cells developing in your body. Yep, you heard me right: bad oils contribute to cancer. If you have never heard this, you either thinking I'm off my rocker or that Peskin is just another guy telling us that everything is bad for us. (Insert exhausted emoji here.) But don't take my word for it. Check out his book *PEO Solutions*. He reviewed thousands of research articles about fish oils to draw these conclusions. Peskin stated that he "feels it's his job to do the research for doctors that do not have the time to put into it." Almost all of the conventional prenatal supplements have fish oil and advertise the presence of DHA in their product. We know preparing our bodies to grow a human requires adequate nutrition, so make sure your prenatal does not contain fish oil. I use a combination organic, plant-based oil supplement that even has a special nitrogen bubble to keep the oils from going rancid.

R3: Restore Cellular Energy

We talked about the importance of a healthy cellular membrane, but did you know we also need to repair the membrane of the mitochondria? Our tiny, little powerhouse cells receive quite a bit more attention these days. We know they produce adenosine triphosphate, or ATP, the energy source for all cellular function. Without adequate production of ATP, our cells cannot detoxify, regenerate, or function properly. If that happens, you will basically feel miserable, and your growing human, even more miserable. It takes a phenomenal amount of energy to grow a human, so in preparing, we cannot overlook the mitochondria.

Nutraceuticals and biohacks can assist in the production of ATP, but that does not mean this is an easy part of the journey. There are many reasons why your cells may not be producing enough ATP and functioning as they should. Viruses, bacteria, previous infections, heavy metals, mold exposures, physical or emotional trauma; all of these play into the speed at which cells heal.

R4: Reduce Inflammation

There are many ways to reduce inflammation. However they may all be in vain if you do not uncover the root problem by removing metals, mold, and hidden infections. I encourage my patients to start with the True Cellular Detox program to address this. Fasting can serve as a very powerful way to reduce inflammation in your cells. We will address fasting in detail as well as fasting while moving through your menstrual cycle in another chapter. If this scares you or turns you off, stay tuned, because we have a strategy to make it not only bearable, but also surprisingly easy in some cases. I've consulted many experts to condense the information to make it as mentally, physically, and emotionally easy as possible. You're welcome!

R5: Reestablish Methylation

This is, by far, my favorite R to discuss, because through the study of epigenetics, we now understand that we can, in fact, change our DNA. You can do more than play the cards you were dealt or wait until you develop a condition common in your family. Put together the five Rs and help your body repair its own DNA. Detoxification, DNA protection, hormone metabolism, and physiological balance all require the presence of methyl groups. Methylation is a natural process occurring in the body and affects the coding of our DNA. That's pretty important considering DNA codes affect every process and function in your body. Toxins and inflammation directly affect methylation, as well as stress and our gut bacteria. Since all these things impact our DNA and we cannot avoid it all, we will probably work to repair it the rest of our days. This makes it all the more important to own the five Rs, practice them, and most importantly, teach our children how to walk this same path to live long, healthy lives where they fulfill their potential.

If all this talk of DNA has you thinking about whether you have the MTHFR gene, take hope as I shed a little light on the subject. The National Institutes of Health (NIH) explains MTHFR or methyltetrahydrofolate reductase as a gene important in a chemical reaction involving folate. Many patients' doctors claim that they will have difficulty detoxing or ingesting B vitamins because they have this gene. Without diving too deep down a rabbit hole, let's recognize that methylation is extremely complex. Because our bodies adapt so amazingly, they create many pathways and workarounds. Also, remember that you can possess a specific gene without turning it on, or expressing it. Dr. Nicholas Morgan noted that environmental toxins and what a person ingests count far more than a single gene in the process of methylation.

All in all, appropriate supplementation, nutrition, and groundwork from the previous 4 Rs will set you up for methylating as the healthy human God designed you.

SECTION 3
AIMING FOR OPTIMAL HEALTH

CHAPTER 4
ARE YOU HEALTHY ENOUGH TO GROW A HUMAN?

Growing a human makes for a very difficult subject. So many factors and emotions play into deciding when to move forward and try to conceive. Understanding a bit more about your body, hormones, and their relationship to your postpartum experience may cause you concern for your own health as well as that of your future tiny human. So how does one evaluate their level of health?

First, reflect on your history, energy levels, previous toxic exposures, and the regularity of your menstrual cycle. Check out the quiz below for details. You can score yourself for a general view of your readiness. For a more concrete look, pursue some testing. Prioritize blood work analyzing your thyroid numbers as well as glucose and insulin; a Dutch Complete urine test to evaluate sex hormones, cortisol, and adrenal function; and an environmental toxin test. Your thyroid plays an integral role in helping a baby's nervous system develop properly, and as we discussed earlier in The Hormone Dance section, your sex hormones and adrenals factor significantly in your pregnancy, labor and delivery, and postpartum season. This environmental toxin test will empower you to identify your exposure to numerous toxins, while providing a starting point for eliminating the highest ones in your environment.

As a physician, I find it very frustrating when a patient says, "Oh, I had my hormones checked and they are fine," and yet see them struggling with energy or immune system issues. Clearly, they are not fine. This patient has typically gone to their obstetrician or another doctor for blood work on their hormones or thyroid. This helps, but it should not serve as our end-all-be-all decision maker. I have two concerns with basing this very important decision on one sheet of blood work results.

First, 95 percent of panels that a general practitioner runs for the thyroid view only T4 and TSH levels. To accurately evaluate your thyroid function, you also need to consider your free T3, T3 uptake, reverse T3, and thyroid antibody levels, and if dysfunction is present, iodine and selenium levels. Just utilizing two of those results will not give you an accurate understanding of your thyroid function. For example, your body may have a normal amount of T4, but it may not be converting T4 to T3, the active hormone that binds to cell receptors to give the cell energy. Also, if you have an abundance of reverse T3, it can block the receptors, preventing T3 from binding and delivering its message into the cell. These are just two examples of legitimate thyroid issues that may not show up on routine blood work.

I have a good friend, a nurse, who works in a hospital and had managed her thyroid challenges for more than fifteen years without a full thyroid panel. Although doctors monitored her T4 and TSH levels, she needed more and more medication every year. Neither she nor her doctors knew *why* her thyroid was not working. She needed more information. When we conducted her blood work, it showed that her antibodies were off the charts. She needed help healing her immune system to ever balance her thyroid. I share her story because she represents thousands of people who need to know there is often more to the story.

Second, if you have inflammation, all of your sex hormones and thyroid numbers can present within normal limits on your blood work, and your doctor may tell you that you are fine; no further investigation is needed. But you still don't feel well, or you have irregular cycles, or you cannot get pregnant. Remember the cell? We know that an inflamed cell membrane cannot function properly.

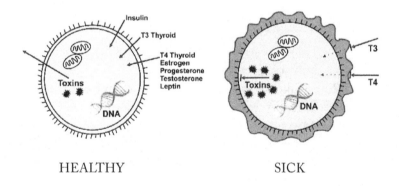

HEALTHY   SICK

Hormones travel through your blood, and for their messages to enter your cells, they have to bind to a receptor located on the cell membrane. With inflamed membranes, hormones cannot bind to the receptors and signal the cell to carry out its needed action. You will have a false sense that everything is "normal," even without properly functioning cells, and in time, organs and systems will not function properly. If you really want a good look at how well your hormones are functioning throughout the day and month, use the Dutch Complete Test, a twenty-four-hour dried-urine test.

Are You Healthy Enough to Grow a Human?
Circle the number that best represents your last six to twelve months.

1. On most days,
    1. I am fatigued and feel sick.
    2. I am tired and depleted, but I have some good days.
    3. I think it's a toss-up. I feel like myself about half of the time.
    4. I feel invincible. I have few low energy days.
    5. I am super woman, and I can do anything I want, anytime I want.

2. Sleep
    1. I sleep restlessly, wake up throughout the night, and wake up tired.
    2. I wake up in the night but go right back to sleep.
    3. I sleep restlessly but don't wake up.
    4. Most days I wake up rested, and some days I feel tired.
    5. I wake up rested and ready to go.

3. Energy
    1. It is hard to get off the couch.
    2. I have more bad days than good.
    3. I am energized for basics but not much past that.
    4. On most days I am the Energizer Bunny, but I do have some rough days.
    5. I am the Energizer Bunny.

4. Exercise
    1. I don't exercise, but when I do, it tanks my energy for the day.
    2. I need a short rest, and then I'm okay.
    3. Exercise has no effect on the rest of my day.
    4. Sometimes exercise energizes me, and sometimes it drains me.
    5. Exercise energizes me for the day.

5. Anxiety
    1. It is daily, constant, and debilitating.
    2. It is constant, but I have some good days.
    3. Only specific situations cause anxiety.
    4. Anxiety is occasional, but I can reframe it and cope.
    5. Hakuna Matata (i.e., no worries).

6. Menstrual Cycle
    1. I am on a form of birth control, or I have debilitating cramping, heavy flow, and PMS.
    2. My period is sporadic; I never know when to expect it.
    3. Every couple of months my period is on time, but with cramps and irritability.
    4. My period is consistent, but I still have cramping and moodiness.
    5. My period is very consistent, five days or fewer of bleeding, and minimal PMS.

Add up your score _____.
Answer the following Yes/No questions, and for every Yes answer, subtract one point from your original score.

1. Has a doctor ever diagnosed you with or suspected you of having mononucleosis or the Epstein-Barr Virus?
2. Have you ever received a flu shot?
3. Were you vaccinated as a child?
4. Do you have amalgam/silver fillings?
5. Do you have any root canals?
6. Do you use personal care products that contain sulfates and parabens?
7. Have you taken any form of birth control?
8. Do you consistently feel overwhelmed or fearful?
9. Have you struggled to conceive or had a miscarriage?
10. Has a doctor ever diagnosed you with or suspected you of having Lyme Disease?
11. Has a doctor ever diagnosed you with or suspected you of having cancer?

Results

0–14 High Toxicity—You have a bit of prep work to do. The True Cellular Detox program will significantly help. However, you also may need a coach to navigate certain protocols such as removing fillings or finding hidden infections. Testing for hormones, thyroid function, and toxicity would be in your best interest. We have many of these resources in the back section of this book.

15–23 Moderate Toxicity—Repairing your foundation as an essential part of your journey. True Cellular Detox will help you clean up years of toxicity and improve your health trajectory. I recommend the Environmental Toxins test as well as evaluating and eliminating the toxins in your daily environment.

24–30 Average Toxicity—You have made your health a priority and have done a good job supporting your body. You may find it easy to work through True Cellular Detox so you can confidently grow your human. Maintaining awareness of the toxins you can eliminate in your daily routine and incorporating physical and emotional healing strategies will benefit you on this journey.

** These results are generalized and cannot compare to a full consultation, as personal history and other factors must be considered in the pursuit of full health.

Example of a checklist (levels correlate with your health history rather than your quiz score):

Base Level

- True Cellular Detox

- Removal of as many toxins from your environment as possible
- Chiropractic care to allow the nervous system to coordinate healing in your body

Next Level

- Dutch Complete test for hormones and adrenal function
- Have amalgams removed by a SMART-certified dentist
- Test your toxic load with the Environmental Toxins test

Deeper Level if needed (includes all of the above)

- Test for Lyme
- Test for autoimmune conditions
- Heavy metal testing with a provoked-urine challenge

CHAPTER 5
REPAIRING YOUR FOUNDATION

Have you or someone you know experienced an emotional trauma such as a difficult divorce or loss of a loved one, and all of the sudden chronic pain, thyroid, or other organ issues appeared? Have you or someone you know undergone physical trauma such as a car accident or sporting injury, and soon after other health problems popped up? In my practice, I often stories like this: "Ever since my epidural fifteen years ago, I have had low back pain," or "Ever since my MRI with contrast (a very toxic drug that lights up specific parts of the images), I have had chronic fatigue," or "I have not been able to sleep well since I had surgery to extract my wisdom teeth." These examples represent chemical trauma to your body.

Healing tools for Physical, Emotional, and Chemical Stresses

Our cells and DNA store trauma, and our bodies do not discriminate between physical, chemical, and emotional trauma. So, in order to fully heal and be our best selves, we must address each of these. Maybe you feel great and have zero health challenges right now, but you know now after reading about heavy metals, mold, and toxins that you carry chemical stress in your body. Maybe you have experienced physical trauma or know that you carry stress in your shoulders or back. Sadly, many of our histories contain emotional trauma. The union of these stresses challenges our health, or even causes it to fail. This could occur, for example, if your history involves chemical or physical stress, then you encounter emotional stress. Likewise, it can occur in the opposite case of a history of emotional stress combined with physical trauma.

Regardless of the trauma you've experienced, I offer practical tools for their healing, as they affect the very foundation of our health.

Physical Tools

Chiropractic

When a patient has struggled with pregnancy or has previously needed intervention to get pregnant starts getting adjusted regularly and out of the blue becomes pregnant, I do a pretty great happy dance. Some of my patients have this running joke: "My chiropractor got me pregnant!" A surprised look usually follows, and then a funny explanation clarifies the matter. It is beautiful to see how the removal of subluxations allows the body to function as it was created to. A subluxation involves a misalignment of one or more bones that causes pressure on the nervous system, and chiropractors specifically train to detect and correct them. They use many techniques in the effort, all gentle and effective, and, in my opinion, essential!

Here's some basic anatomy for you. Our nervous system controls and runs everything in the entire body. God designed the spine to move, but also to protect that very delicate nervous system. Subluxations or misalignments in the spine or joints affect the nerve at that location, decreasing the function of the tissue or organ system connected to the nerve that carries signals back and forth. The base of your spine, your sacrum, connects to the pelvis and the iliac bones. The uterus sits in the pelvis and connects to those bones by ligaments. That delicate relationship is instrumental in allowing a baby to develop while in the proper position. When a woman gets adjusted throughout pregnancy, she can ensure that her pelvis sits in the most balanced position. This allows for babies to drop, turn, and rotate as they need to throughout the growth and labor process. Many forces act on the position of the pelvis including bone position. Ligaments, muscles, fascia, previous trauma, inflammation, and many other physical stressors also act upon it.

The Webster Technique is a specific assessment and adjustment during the third trimester that focuses on the alignment of the pelvis as well as the ligaments in the front of the belly. Many women come to our office because their babies are breech, posterior, or in other malpositions, and we can to use this specific technique to support the baby by turning it to a birth-ready, head-down position. This is a much gentler technique than the medical version of turning a baby. Instead of forcing the movement, this technique puts the mother's body in proper alignment and allows the baby to move into the proper position on its own. Some women report feeling a mini "earthquake" in the middle of the night after having their first Webster adjustment, when the baby turned on its own.

A chiropractic adjustment removes interference in the nervous system, which improves the function of the mother's body even to a cellular level. This reflects the great importance of chiropractic care in preparing your body to grow a human. Remember, our organs do not operate independently. They connect at an intricate level. We can observe how an adjustment improves the body's ability to digest, assimilate, and absorb nutrients, which affects brain chemistry, hormones, as well as our response to our environment. We call this beautiful symphony of function *innate intelligence.* You and all your tiny humans-to-be will have this programmed into them from conception. Chiropractic care is foundational and essential to all humans who wish to have a strong and healthy spine and nervous system. Let's continue the journey of finding and removing any interference to our body's ability to heal and function.

> **Remember, our organs do not operate independently. They connect at an intricate level.**

I personally don't know how anyone could make it through pregnancy without getting adjusted. I was adjusted every week of my pregnancy—and multiple times a week in the last two months. Now as a chiropractor who's married to a chiropractor, this may sound easier said than done. However, people wildly underestimate the value of chiropractic adjustment, which needs more awareness and understanding. I believe if people fully understood the benefit of it, they would see it as a complete no-brainer, no-questions-asked, do-whatever-it-takes-to-make-it-happen goal.

Many midwives will not accept a patient unless they agree to chiropractic care throughout pregnancy. Now that is a testimony, if I have ever heard one. Midwives have the opportunity to see firsthand how a well-adjusted mama experiences decreased labor time and complications. Yahoo for that! Many of my patients who have had multiple pregnancies experienced similar results. They found that chiropractic during successive pregnancies equated to less pain, decreased labor times, and minimal pushing.

In my practice, I've taken care of many different women with many unique experiences. Some bounce into the office at thirty-eight and even forty-two weeks of pregnancy with no pain—loving life and loving pregnancy. We adjust them, keep them balanced, and help them feel amazing. They usually push for twenty minutes before their babies enter the world. On the opposite side, some women experience every day as a struggle, with low back pain or pubic bone pain that makes daily tasks seem impossible. I love the privilege of journeying with these women. Many skilled chiropractors care for ladies during pregnancy; to find a Webster-certified doc near you, use this great resource at icpa4kids.org.

Massage

One highly specific massage technique focuses directly on fertility and preparing your body to grow a human. It uses foot reflexology and abdominal castor oil packs, with application during a specific window of the menstrual cycle. Therapists massage you lower back and abdomen gently repositioning the uterus. This may sound scary, but it is a very light technique that can decrease cramping, clotting, and bleeding time during your cycle. I have a friend trained in this technique, and I send people to her when they are ready to get pregnant. It also greatly benefits inflammatory conditions of the ovaries or uterus, like PCOS or endometriosis, and provides support for irregular cycling. I personally have had several of these massages and experienced a smoother cycle the following month.

If I could get a massage every week, I would be a happy camper. It's not just the hour of turning off my cell phone, disconnecting, and relaxing. It's the sheer fact that the benefits of massage go far deeper than just releasing muscle tension and relaxing your brain. Having your fascia stretched and massaged helps correct altered motor patterns, assists in the movement of lymph, increases blood flow to tissue, and even helps push toxins out of tissues so our bodies can properly eliminate them. Massage therapists trained in medical massage perform stretching that helps with dysfunction in your fascia.

If you are, in fact, trying to keep your pelvis in the most optimal position, you need some type of massage or soft-tissue work. This plays a crucial role in stabilizing chiropractic adjustments and strengthening your body so you can push out a human.

Anytime you're injured, your body acts to heal itself. Swelling protects the injured area, and increased blood flow shows up as redness and heat. Then, your body creates a protective mechanism where different muscles compensate to give the injured area a break. This workaround creates altered motor patterns, and if not properly rested and healed, they can lead to dysfunction. Have you noticed painful trigger points on your body? Knots in your shoulders or glutes? These evidence problems that chiropractic care and massage can address, to assist your healing. Without further ado, get on the phone and schedule yourself a massage appointment.

Craniosacral Therapy

Craniosacral therapy or CST is a very light-touch therapeutic massage that helps to balance and calm the central nervous system. When you encounter stress, your sympathetic nervous system jumps in the driver's seat as it handles your fight-or-flight responses. It is then meant to turn off as the parasympathetic nervous system takes over. This rest-and-digest system should assume control the majority of the time, as all healing functions happen in this state. What happens when we experience stress all day long, every day, though? Our sympathetic nervous system gets stuck in overdrive, and disease originates or worsens. When this happens, you need to pull out your toolbox and find a good CST practitioner. (Check out the resources in the back of this book.)

Note: Do not wait until you are stuck in a sympathetic state. Consider adding CST to your monthly routine to prevent your nervous system from imbalance. I personally do my best to have CST every three to four weeks, because that is what my body needs. When I'm done, I walk out of that room feeling more like myself, ready to take on the world.

Every cell in your body has memory. Cells can hold trauma, stress, or tension, and treatments of CST with mindfulness can help release that energy from your body. This allows you to move forward and heal even events that you might not remember. We don't remember this, but we felt our own birth process as well as our mother's experience of our birth. As you grow a healthy human, you might want to release any trauma or negative emotions that you might unknowingly carry into your own delivery story.

Craniosacral therapy helps you communicate with your body, important for many reasons, but even more important as you endeavor to carry a tiny human in your body. Some people naturally listen to their bodies, but some of us really have to work at learning to listen. God gave us all amazing innate intelligence. This intuition is meant for our own healing as well as a means of knowing what our baby needs before they even ask (or cry, in the case of an infant). Listen to and trust your "mama gut." It will be the best tool you have as a mother. Tap into it now through loving and supporting yourself as you prepare to grow a healthy human.

> Listen to and trust your "mama gut." It will be the best tool you have as a mother.

When CST is performed during pregnancy, babies benefit because they feel everything you do. You share energy with one another. Therapists spend intentional time balancing the temporal bones and jaw muscles, which are instrumental in a balanced pelvis. When you are near the time of delivery, CST releases the coccyx amazingly and helps the pelvic floor muscles relax, for a safer, and hopefully faster, delivery.

I could not be prouder to tell you that I learned many of these concepts from my mother. While I was in chiropractic school, she and my dad became empty nesters as my youngest brother moved away to college. She then went to massage school and discovered that she loved cranial work. She poured hours into seminars and trainings, even after school. She now works in our office, and I feel so blessed that with chiropractic adjustments and CST together, women and their babies are experiencing healing on multiple levels. Shout out to all the mamas following their calling at any and all times in their lives!

Loving on Your Lymph System

The lymphatic system filters bacteria, viruses, and dead cells; it also produces lymphocytes to fight infection. You might notice this system working when you have a cold and your neck feels sore and swollen. Your lymph nodes are doing their job.

Do you know that lymph makes up two-thirds of your body, yet most medical textbooks give it little attention? It's overlooked and underestimated, but we know that your lymph directly connects with your immune system and fascia. It is instrumental in helping us to remove toxins. Your body cannot eliminate toxins with a stagnant lymph system. Life constantly exposes us to toxins, so we vitally and continually need to support the lymph system so it moves and functions properly.

Experts advise us to do so many things to stay healthy—exercise, drink water, balance our electrolytes. Do you know that every one of these things impacts your lymph system? Check your lymph movement by looking at your armpits. Yes, I said armpits. Do they look like "pits" or "puffs"?

After having my son and nursing, I maintained my pregnancy weight. I didn't like my upper body, especially my armpits. I felt bloated and puffy—I just figured I wasn't exercising enough. At one of our "Live It to Lead It" seminars, Kelly Kennedy spoke to our Platinum group about lymph. She possesses a wealth of knowledge after training for the last twenty years in Europe and New Zealand with many types of doctors. I will never forget her lifting her arm on stage while wearing a tank top. She asked us all, "Do you have pits or puffs under your arms?" The puffs indicate a sluggish lymph system. It was a relief to know that I was not simply chubby. My armpit puffs formed for a reason, and I could do something to fix it. Now even if you do have nice armpits (that sounds so funny) it still is important to intentionally work on moving your lymph.

Here are a few tools you can work into your weekly routine to keep your lymph flowing. When I feel my immune system struggling or I engage in detoxification, I make sure to use as many of these tools as I can.

- Lymph pumping—light pressure pumping action of specific sites on your body with the intention of moving your lymph. Download in Resources Section.

- Dry brushing—this simple yet effective tool moves your lymph. It seems too simple to work (but my armpits prove that it does). Learn the right versus wrong way to dry brush; the description below will ensure your success.

- Rebounding—time to bust out that little mini trampoline that has been collecting dust in the basement. Just a few minutes a day bouncing up and down can get your lymph flowing and provide many other benefits.

- Vibration plates—Vibration therapy will help move your lymph, increase bone density, and reset your postural muscles. Find these at chiropractic offices, wellness centers, and gyms, although you can purchase a great home unit for around $300.

- Balancing your electrolytes—make sure you have quality minerals like magnesium, calcium, and potassium in your diet or supplements, as well as good salt. No low quality, processed salt.

- Massage—A therapist specifically trained in lymph massage would be my first choice, but any massage is going to benefit the lymph system.

- Yoga—Stretching your fascia is so productive as it aids in the flow of lymph. Some yoga positions open channels for your lymph to flow more efficiently.

- FLOWpresso sessions—These may be hard to find, but I use this new equipment in our office. Far-infrared heat with grounding technology and whole-body light compression cyclically moves lymph. Word is getting out, so you may find an office near you that offers it. Good luck—it's amazing!

Kennedy gave this analogy to help us properly dry brush and pump our lymph. Picture your lymph system as several highways. A tollbooth sits right above your left clavicle. You have roads full of cars all down your arms and legs. If this tollbooth backs up, nothing moves. You must open the tollbooth before any cars can get through it. You also must move the closest car to the tollbooth before you can move the fifty cars down your arms and the one hundred cars down your legs. You want to move everything toward your heart and the cisterna chyli, one of the larger lymph nodes located below your sternum. Dry brushing and pumping in that fashion will give you the most bang for your buck. Adding some flow cream, balancing your electrolytes, and doing some old-fashioned stretching will really take you far in this piece of the puzzle. Kennedy has a great resource teaching you about lymph pumping on her website, www.notmeds.com.

The fascia also affects your lymph's ability to move. Fascia is thin sheath that surrounds your entire body, underneath your skin. Have you ever deboned a chicken or some other form of meat? A cellophane-like sheath lies just beneath the skin called the *fascia*. It contains so many important components that medical textbooks now contain chapters about it. All of these components affect your musculoskeletal system, the flow of your lymph, and your ability to detoxify on a daily basis. Like muscles, fascia has memory and can change with injuries. With lack of movement or trauma, it can tighten or even physically shorten.

Acupuncture

In the last year I have been regularly getting acupuncture. I cannot believe I waited so long. It not only relaxes, but facilitates detoxification, opening up energy channels and supporting overall health. I recommend starting acupuncture at least three to four months before trying to conceive. However, you can utilize it at any stage of the fertility process. My interview with Dr. Ashley Marcheck Vincen will be available in the Growing Healthy Humans membership site where she lays out when to get started and explains what to expect at your first acupuncture. Dr. Ashley is one of those amazing people that went to school to be a doctor and then could not stop learning, accomplishing two diplomas and a fellowship in acupuncture. Honestly, I was nervous for my first one, but she made it easy and pain free!

Traditional Chinese doctors consider infertility a disruption in balance between qi (energy) and blood circulation. With disruption, energy and blood do not freely circulate to support and nourish the male and female reproductive organs. Dr. Ashley explained how the uterus is referred to as "the palace" because that is where your little prince or princess will be grown. This may sound silly, but throughout my acupuncture sessions I would lie there and picture my blood and energy going to my uterus and my whole body healing, preparing my little one's palace. ☺

When you get pregnant, acupuncture can help support you through each trimester as well as the postpartum period. I listed some examples below, complete with my comments and notations.

- **Trimester Zero: Balancing energy to nourish your reproductive organs**

    I love the word *nourish*. With our stressful lives, our bodies can slip into survival mode where less blood flow and nutrients get to the reproductive organs.

- **First Trimester: Fatigue, morning sickness, constipation, headaches, and nausea**

    If you have experienced these symptoms, you would probably do anything in your power to ease them. I am personally excited to use acupuncture the next time I grow a human.

- **Second Trimester: Heartburn, edema, hemorrhoids, back pain, and high blood pressure**

    Consider how each of these symptoms reflects a struggling system. Use acupuncture to prevent and relieve them.

- **Third Trimester: Back and pelvic pain, breeched position, and inducing labor when it's time**

    Remembering the amazing symphony of hormones that initiate labor gives me a new respect for my body. Knowing that acupuncture can aid in this natural process provides hope and affirmation that I am doing something great for myself and my baby.

- **Fourth Trimester, Postpartum: Poor milk supply, fatigue, mood (anxiety or depression)**

    Recognize the intricacies of your body's response to stress on a physical, emotional, and chemical level. Supporting energy channels that help with healing and adaptation could be a game changer for you! Add this excellent tool to your regimen of preparing your body to grow a human.

Fasting for Hormone Balance

As we work with patients on their healing journey, we incorporate as many healing strategies as we can, but those who see the fastest and best results embrace fasting. God designed humans for seasons of feast and famine. With these fasting strategies, you will soon be saying, "That was easier than I thought." Understand that fasting does not equal starving! If you have PCOS, endometriosis, abnormal periods, or weight loss resistance, this section will be your best friend. If you already feel awesome, this will be an amazing way to optimize your hormones and set you up for a healthy pregnancy and postpartum season. Lastly, if you get shaky or lightheaded when you don't eat, do *not* disqualify yourself from this opportunity. These strategies are built for you, my friend.

> Fasting does not equal starving!

When most people prepare to grow a tiny human, they don't place fasting at the top of their to-do list. It is, however, vitally important to balance your hormones and understand how insulin influences your sex hormones: estrogen, progesterone, and testosterone. What's the best way to control insulin? Controlling not only *what* you eat, but *when* you eat it. In other words, intermittent fasting, most effective when combined with a keto diet of good fats and fewer processed carbohydrates (more details later in the book). *Keto* or *ketogenic* comes from the word *ketone*, which fuels your body (in preference to glucose) and is a byproduct of your body burning fats. Therefore, a keto diet involves selecting foods that help your body burn more fat and less glucose.

I interviewed Dr. Mindy Pelz, who has built a community of more than 350,000 people fasting together to regain their health. With a fun and direct style, she teaches people how to fast properly and balance their hormones during perimenopause. She is passionate about fasting, and I feel blessed to pick her brain for all of you. After you read this book, check out our interview on our *Growing Healthy Humans* You Tube channel.

Dr. Pelz clearly explains the best times to fast or feast during our monthly cycle. Combining a clean keto approach with the strategies of intermittent fasting can make you more sensitive to insulin, and in turn keep it in check to help balance your sex hormones. I truly believe it is an art to listen to your body and what it needs. These strategies enable you to do that, and to understand the difference between feeling hungry and actually needing nutrients.

Our cells need to flex between burning glucose or ketones for fuel. This promotes healing and longevity, but it only happens through cycling feast and famine times. Intermittent fasting is where you extend your "breakfast" time later into the afternoon and you keep all your eating in a "window." Block fasting is where you fast for 24 hours or more just having water or possibly coffee. It might seem that men have an easier time fasting or lose weight faster. However, if you lean into your cycle and listen to your body, I believe we have an advantage. It's certainly not a competition, but I want to give you a little ray of hope.

Let's explore the menstrual cycle. We will discuss your body's needs related to food and throw in some exercise advice. First, though, we need to track your cycle. So many free apps exist for this; pick one and start entering data. Basal body temperature and ovulation strips will substantially help as well.

Call Day One the day you start your period. This is a very important time to balance your body's response to insulin. That means intermittent fasting or even block fasting is okay at this time. Many women find this time the easiest to fast, **if** they nurtured themselves well the week before. Cardio or high-intensity interval training (HIIT) also works well during this time if your body can handle working out.

Ovulation usually occurs between day twelve and day fourteen, and at this point, you're going to need more insulin so add in those good complex carbohydrates. Your sex hormones are in a good place here, so you usually feel your best. Strength training is most productive during this time. Don't be surprised if you feel hungrier. Listen to your body and eat healthy, organic fats and complex carbs like quinoa and lentils.

After ovulation, between day fourteen and day twenty-one, you can water fast or intermittent fast. This again is a good time for cardio, or to push yourself a bit.

On day twenty-one until you start your period, you're making progesterone and will need more good carbohydrates, seeds, squash, beans, rice, sweet potatoes, and the like to start the cycle all over again. This is an important time to nurture your body and prepare for menstruation. Activities such as yoga, walking, or less intense exercise will help you make the most of this week (or so). I personally have a calendar I use just for health habits inside my supplement cupboard, where I record when to fast and feast. When I wake up in the morning, I can set my intentions for the day.

Let's recap:
Day One to Day Twelve = Intermittent and block fasting, cardio or HIIT workouts
Day Twelve to Day Fourteen = Add complex carbs, strength training is productive here
Day Fourteen to Day Twenty-One = Intermittent fasting and more intense workouts allowed
Day Twenty-One to Period Start = Nurture, quality foods, yoga or walking is best here

Let's tap back into the topic of hormone resistance. (Refer back to the Are You Healthy Enough to Grow a Human section for more detail.) Even when all of the hormones in your body are at appropriate levels, inflammation of the cellular membrane can still keep them from fully binding with receptors to get their messages into the cell. How do your cell membranes become inflamed? It happens when we simply eat, drink, or breathe anywhere on this planet. That might sound a bit dramatic, but we're living in the most toxic time known to humans, and these toxins affect our cell and mitochondrial membranes. With tragic consequences, only specific healing and detox strategies will help us move beyond these problems.

> We're living in the most toxic time known to humans, and these toxins affect our cell and mitochondrial membranes.

Once you learn and apply these fasting principles at the appropriate time during your cycle, watch your brain get sharper, your PMS symptoms lessen, and probably even your frame drop a few pounds, because fasting also downregulates inflammation. If in fact you feel better, you will most likely notice a healthy change in your relationships. Not only are you worth it, but you have nothing to lose if you try! Remember, healing takes time, so give it a few months and be patient with yourself. Then teach your family this lost art of fasting!

Detoxing alone may not help you achieve all your health goals. That's why we have to incorporate seasons of feast and famine, as well as diet variation. When Dr. Pompa started teaching our Platinum group about this, I was so excited to learn principles that respect the uniqueness of individuals. No diet will fix everyone, and no health strategy will yield a one-size-fits-all result.

Every time I hear different perspectives on health or diet, they mostly present a singular view of

> No health strategy will yield a one-size-fits-all result.

how the world needs to eat to save the human race. Many seemed a bit narrow minded, unable consider every side of the issue. In reality, many paths to optimal health exist. We need to eat with the seasons and consistently vary our food choices. We might need to eat keto for a little while, then incorporate more fruits and vegetables, and seasonal seeds and nuts. Limiting ourselves to vegetables or even short periods of a carnivorous diet can produce extremely effective results in resetting our microbiome. It makes beautiful sense to rotate our nutrients as our bodies are complex and need many different things.

For a deeper understanding on these topics, I recommend three books. First, *Beyond Fasting* by Dr. Dan Pompa. He gives you week-by-week instructions on how to fast with the intention of healing your body at a cellular level. Second, *Eat, Fast, Feast* by pastor Jay Richards. Richards' book guides Christians in fasting, providing a detailed understanding of fasting (and its spiritual benefits), intermittent fasting, and feasting. Coming in 2021, Dr Mindy Pelz will launch a book that outlines fasting for your menstrual cycle, so you can share it with all of your friends. But for now, you got the inside scoop straight from the author!

Emotional Tools

In early spring, 2020, my husband and I were ready to try to conceive. I had weaned my son the previous year and used fasting and detox to ready my body for another baby. In March, 2020, I saw a full picture of stress's impact on health. The declared "pandemic" suffocated us, shutting down businesses, establishing widespread restrictions, and fostering feelings of impending doom. I am sure many of you shared these experiences. So much changed, and stressful situations driven by fear seemed to lurk around every corner. We had to make tough business decisions and stand against the crowd in many situations. Frankly, I had a hard time keeping my peace. The thought even creeped into my mind of *why would I want to bring a child into this world as it is*. Navigating these changes for my family was my first priority, but I still felt a burning responsibility to dive past censorship and get the real facts for my patients as a leader in my community. Needless to say I felt stressed on a new level.

In April, I decided to run a Dutch Complete test to evaluate my hormones, adrenals, and cortisol levels to make sure they were optimal to grow a human. Much to my dismay, my progesterone had tanked, my estrogen had skyrocketed, and my cortisol had sunk so low that feeling drained every day actually made sense. My hormones looked exactly the opposite the year before. I knew that if I got pregnant right away, without enough progesterone, I would more than likely miscarry. I had no idea how quickly stress could affect my hormones until I saw it in full color on my Dutch Complete report.

Fortunately, over the past few years, Dr. Sonya Jensen has helped me navigate my healing process. (Even doctors need doctors!) She and her husband, both naturopathic doctors, own a wellness center in Vancouver, Canada. They have extensive training in women's health. Dr. Jensen is passionate about helping women find true healing, so they truly thrive rather than survive. I can think of many times I slipped into surviving rather than thriving, and I can see how stress drove me to it. Dr. Jensen reflects on our body's response to stress. Much of this section presents a transcription of our interview, so you can get the most out of the conversation we had.

I asked Dr. Jenson how stress affects our hormones, and this is the beautiful description she gave me:

> Stress is the number one thing that is going to influence how our body is responding to life. And with women, our hormonal system is so intricate that it's always on the lookout—watching, guarding, and communicating. So I think one misconception that a lot of women have is that

the hormone is a result. But really, the hormone is taking information from an input and giving it to a cell so that the body can respond appropriately with the input that it's getting. So if it's getting an input of stress, and that could be anything from a car accident, to something that happened in your childhood, to a conversation with your partner that just isn't working out that day, your body and your mind do everything they can to help you survive.

So the first thing that's going to happen is your amygdala gets activated. It then takes information from your hippocampus, which is your memory center. It then is looking into your limbic system, which is your emotional center. And then an emotion is evoked, and then from there, it's going to contact your pituitary to say, "Hey, I've got some stress going on; give me the hormones. I need to deal with this stress right now, in this moment." And more often than not, the hormones that get released are cortisol and adrenaline. And when cortisol is high in our body, we're kind of stuck in a state of surviving rather than thriving. But when we look at a woman's hormonal system, we have estrogen, progesterone, testosterone, we have the DHEA, we have all these hormones that help regulate our everyday functions, regulate our cycle. They get us prepared for pregnancy. Progesterone is very specific in that regulation process and is converted into cortisol every time you need it. Therefore, in a state of constant stress progesterone will be depleted, and you cannot carry a pregnancy without progesterone.

If you imagine walking through life, even [in one] as young as a three-year-old, the hormonal system is starting to wake up. And all of that time, if we're experiencing stress, our progesterone is continuously pouring itself into cortisol, just to keep us alive. And again, depending on our perception of the event, because we're all going to have stress; that is inevitable as the world is always changing. Uncertainty is in the air all the time. But it's how we receive the information that then the hormones will figure out, "What do I need to do with this? And what signal do I need to give the body to react or to respond?" That's kind of like the big picture of how stress can really influence how we're navigating through life.

What's a girl to do?

The Power of a Reframe

Dr. Sonya also shared an example of her son going through a traumatic experience.

> We moved last year, and this was a very traumatic event for my eight-year-old son. He felt his whole world was crumbling: to lose the only home he has ever lived in, lose his friends. All of that was where life was. And now we uprooted him and brought him to another place, which is bigger. There's more space for him and his brother to play; we're closer to our family. There were many benefits, but to him, his world was ending because of a move. His reaction was a lot of anger. He also went more internal and going from the guy that was a leader in his group and his classroom to somebody really shy and now having challenges with reading and other things at school. So my first reaction as a mom was, I just wanted to cover him and protect him and take the pain away. And then I had to really step back and recognize that I am putting my own reactions in my body onto him, and my expectations. So what I did with him one day when he was so angry, I said, "Okay, we're going to be angry together, because what you're feeling is real."
>
> I think a lot of times what happens is, when we have these signals from our emotions, I call them our senses of our soul, they give us an opportunity to recognize what's happening. If we suppress the emotion, the hormones are going to pack this up into my memory. Then when I

have this emotion again, my brain says I'm supposed to suppress, not express. So then I gave him an opportunity to be angry. I followed his lead, and we were punching the pillows, we were screaming, and we were kicking. After he had a safe space to experience and express his emotions, then we were able to have a conversation. We were able to reframe, and then I was able to share with him, "Look at this from this perspective. You had friends in this one city; now you're going to have friends here, so you have more friends now. Nothing was taken away. If anything we're adding to your life."

As humans, we're so used to looking at what's not working and what we've had to give up, that we forget what we're gaining in that moment. So we have to reframe things. I asked my son, "What is working for you at school? What's working for you in this home? What do you like about here? And what are you grieving? What do you miss about over there? What can we do to maybe incorporate some of that over here?"

I found the more questions I asked him, the easier it was for him to recognize, *Okay, I can shift this.*

But if I say, "Hey, you should be grateful that we have a bigger home now," it's taking their experience away, and it's not acknowledging that what he is feeling is valid and real for him. It could be something as simple as losing a Lego piece that was so priceless to him. To us, it's just a silly Lego. Right? But to him, *"It's my whole world and it can't continue without this Lego! And you're not acknowledging my feelings."*

Fast forward twenty years. What if he's in a relationship and needs something. If he doesn't ask, because he assumes his feelings won't get acknowledged, well, now now my response from twenty years earlier affects their relationship.

Listening to her story, I first thought of her as a great mom. Then, as I tried to apply those strategies to a situation of my own, it occurred to me. I sometimes do not allow myself the time or the space to really experience my emotions. I certainly want to create safe spaces for my children to experience and reframe their emotions, so why do I not extend the same grace to myself? Our perception of an event largely determines whether we react or respond. So maybe to decrease our everyday stress, we need to start asking ourselves more questions. We then would respond more than react. Like us all, I am a work in progress, but this last year I determined to set boundaries for myself so that I do not get overwhelmed. Of course, I still get overwhelmed sometimes, but if I want to show up as my best self for my loved ones, I have to take care of myself. I love the way Dr. Sonya referred to her important practices as *nonnegotiables*. Maybe you could take a few minutes and write out yours. Check out the rest of our interview on YouTube if you want to hear more from Dr. Sonya and look for her new book early 2022, *Woman Unleashed*.

> Our perception of an event largely determines whether we react or respond.

Action Steps

1. Ask yourself more questions. Allow yourself a safe space to process and reframe situations.
2. Set your nonnegotiables.

Other Tools for Emotional Support

Reading, journaling, prayers, or gratitude
Yoga and meditation
Tapping

Practitioner-led Tools

Neuro-Emotional Technique
Emotional Freedom Technique
Somato-Emotional Release
Eye Movement Desensitization and Reprocessing (EMDR)
Craniosacral Therapy

Setting Up Your Child's Emotional Success

Mothers have the unique position and responsibility of shaping how their babies feel about themselves as well as how they view relationships throughout their lives. This sobering fact slapped me in the face, then gave me a profound sense of responsibility that changed and deepened how I love my son. Brenda Hunter does an amazing job describing it in her book *The Power of Mother Love*. I encourage you to read it. That statement may have made you feel warm and fuzzy, or it may have hit you in the pit of your stomach with a nice combination of fear, pain, and sheer overwhelm. No matter what you felt, I believe healing and peace are available for those who seek! I recommend that every daughter who wants to grow as a mother read her book. It gave me powerful understanding that in each season as mothers, we have a unique opportunity to heal the childhood wounds in our soul. It also allowed me to extend grace for my own shortcomings and be more at peace with myself. I personally affirm myself multiple times a day by saying, "God chose me to be Titus's mommy, knowing fully my strengths *and* my weaknesses."

This blurb appears on the back cover of her book. I added it here to entice you to read it for yourself.

> *Mother love shapes cultures and individuals. While most mothers know that their love and emotional availability are vital to their children's well-being, many of us do not understand the profound and long-lasting impact we have in developing our young children's brains, teaching them first lessons of love, shaping their consciences . . . At a time when society urges women to seek their worth and personal fulfillment in things that take them away from their families and intimate bonds, Hunter invites women to come home—to their children, their best selves, their hearts.*

From *The Power of Mother Love* by Brenda Hunter, PhD

Chemical Tools

Prenatal Supplements

What would a book about pregnancy prep be without a section on prenatal supplements? I could probably sum up my best recommendation in one sentence, so here it is: not all supplements are created equally, so know what you are putting in your body. So many manufacturers synthetically source their supplements, and not only do they fail to act as promised in your body, they also can create inflammation. This happens even with prenatal vitamins prescribed by physicians, so do your homework and find out what makes up that little capsule! Take a look at the "extra ingredients" on the label. If you see soybean oil, dextrose, or other questionable ingredients, pitch it. (I'll list specific brands in the resource section.) Refer back to the section on repairing the cell membrane for a detailed explanation of why you should avoid fish oil (or any other rancid oil).

Look for whole-food supplements, as research shows you will absorb far more of the nutrients. Do you know there are more than six thousand enzymes in an apple? You can't get that kind of nutrition by simply taking vitamins A, B, C, or D. You need the whole food.

A Note on Essential Oils

Essential oils are an amazing tool for supporting the body chemically, physically, and emotionally. For hundreds of years, people have used plants for healing, and I like to think of them as God's little chemicals gifted to us. I have used oils for all kinds of support, but especially throughout my pregnancy. Now, with our little boy, they have been life savers!

Every organ system in your body vibrates at a specific frequency, and we know that many things can throw it off. Oils are the "lifeblood" of the plant, and they also have individual frequencies. When we match them with an appropriate location or appropriate emotion, they have the ability to create balance in the body and aid in the healing process.

Many people and books promote essential oils. I have used these in my journey: *Releasing Emotional Patterns with Essential oils* by Carolyn Mein DC, and *Feelings Buried Alive Never Die* by Karol Truman. For pregnancy and baby resources, I used *Gentle Babies* by Debra Raybern. Most importantly, whether you use oils on your body, in your body, or diffuse them, make sure they are pure and sourced with integrity. Buy organic, from companies with transparent labeling for everything, down to the cleaning of the equipment utilized for harvesting the oils. Third-party testing also demonstrates that no contamination or dilution has occurred with synthetic oils. I highly recommend adding these basic essentials to your medicine cabinet.

I personally use Young Living oils. If you were going to start with just a few, here are my top recommendations that I make sure I never run out of. Tea Tree or Melaleuca, Lavender, Frankincense, Digize or the kids version Tummygize, Seedlings Calm, and my personal savior for much needed baby/toddler nap times... Sleepygize!!! Maybe you should just get online and buy the *Gentle Babies* book right now.

Basic Nutrition Reminders

I will not spend too much time on this topic because so much information about nutrition exists that I don't need to reinvent the wheel. Everybody needs different nutrients. Instead of telling you exactly what you should eat, I would like to lay out my personal nonnegotiables. Check out my list and then build your own plan for preparing your body to grow a human.

First, understand that God didn't design us to adhere to any diet or plan for too long. This is exciting because dietary changes can be difficult, but they don't have to last forever. Now if you still drink diet sodas, that is a different story. You should probably never drink that again if you want to grow a healthy human and stay around long enough to watch them grow up.

Variation in your diet is so important and living in the United States makes that a real challenge. Why? Because we have access to every type of food at all times! It is all too easy to eat the same things all the time—especially after working hard to master a new lifestyle shift. Yes, this means you should *not* "do keto" for the rest of your life. You should, however, give it your best shot if you are trying to optimize your hormones. Couple keto with the fasting strategies discussed in the Physical Tools section of this chapter.

What the Heck Is Keto, Anyway?

I do not know many people who have not heard of the ketogenic diet. If you're like me, though, you're not about to jump on the train of some fad diet. But have no fear my friends, keto is not one of those. Keto is not new. There have been similar low-carb diets (you might remember the popular Atkins diet). For centuries, different civilizations have eaten low-carb/high-fat diets. Contrary to what some would like to believe, this does not grant a free pass to eat bacon and cheddar at every meal. You can eat a clean keto diet, or a dirty one. Guess which one's best for you? Yep, the clean keto. Eating bad fats like canola or vegetable oil will cause inflammation of the cellular membrane and basically negate all your hard work of optimizing your hormones.

Simply observing a ketogenic diet will not fix everything. You also need strategies such as intermittent fasting. Now if you have never tried a ketogenic diet, then I highly recommend you jump on this train. If you have any trouble with your insulin, thyroid hormones, or sex hormones, I believe it is *essential* that you jump on this train. Let me explain why.

Every time you put something in your mouth other than water, your body releases insulin. Insulin drives glucose into your cells, which they need for fuel. But cells can also burn ketones, the by-product fat metabolism, as fuel. Our cells have two options. Because they burn glucose more easily, they will choose glucose first. Without the availability of glucose, our cells will use ketones, which surprisingly function more efficiently, with less toxic waste.

Refer to the picture of a cell, and note that insulin has to bind to a receptor to deliver its message into the cell. You must increase a diabetic's insulin intake over time, because the more you fire insulin into a cell, the more resistant that cell becomes. I would guess the average American eats at least fifteen times a day. Every time you snack on some almonds, eat a granola bar, grab a banana, or even pop a mint or chew a piece of gum, your pancreas has to release insulin. To balance the body's insulin, we must decrease the frequency of releasing it. Right here is where your pancreas breathes a sigh of relief. It's also where intermittent fasting and the ketogenic diet come into play.

The real goal? Teach your cells to burn fat rather than sugar. To do this, you must deprive the cells of glucose so they will look for fat. This is possibly when you may feel shaky or lightheaded and the solution is to eat good fats. By eating fewer carbs along with adequate, quality fat, you can train your mitochondria to burn ketones instead of glucose. Aim for metabolic flexibility, where your cells can burn one or the other. To reap the full benefits of a ketogenic diet, the timing must be right.

Picture a large, gas tanker truck that runs out of gas on its way to refill at the local gas station. Isn't that ironic? This giant truck, filled with gasoline, sits stuck on the side of the road because of an empty fuel tank. That is similar to our bodies! Have you ever felt like you had extra fat, but couldn't burn it by going to the gym or climbing every flight of stairs possible? We actually have to train our bodies to burn fat. This book is not about weight loss, but it's important and helpful to understand that weight-loss resistance is actually a hormonal issue. In the smallest nutshell possible, keto involves taking in moderate protein, increasing good fats, eliminating bad fats, and keeping net carbs to roughly fifty to seventy grams a day. Those numbers will fluctuate, of course, depending on your activity level or if you are pregnant or nursing.

Weight-loss resistance is actually a hormonal issue.

Benefits of a Ketogenic Diet with Intermittent Fasting

- Decreased cellular inflammation
- Increased insulin sensitivity
- Clearing of brain fog
- Increased testosterone (yes, this is important for women too)
- Sex hormone optimization (estrogen, progesterone, testosterone, and DHEA)

I personally move in and out of a keto diet every couple of months, but here we finally get to my nonnegotiables. I won't make recommendations for patients I have never seen, but I thought it would be fun to share my diet, and you can implement it as little or as much as you want! We are all in this boat together.

Nonnegotiable	WHY?	Reference for your own research
I do NOT eat wheat	It is genetically modified, contains glyphosate, disrupts gut permeability, creates autoimmune conditions, and worst of all, contains excitotoxins that bind to the receptors in our brain, causing addictive behaviors and altering our brain chemistry.	Read: *Wheat Belly* and *Grain Brain* Watch: the documentary, *What's with Wheat?*
I do NOT eat anything with canola or vegetable oil.	They are bad fats that rapidly create inflammation at a cellular level.	Read: "R2: Regenerate the Cell Membrane" section in Chapter 3 Watch: Dr. Pompa's video on *Regenerating the Membrane* and the documentaries *Fat Fiction* and *The Magic Pill*
I do NOT eat or drink anything containing artificial sweeteners, dyes, or preservatives.	They deteriorate the brain, damage the gut, and cause weight gain.	Watch: *Sweet Misery*
I do NOT eat past 8:00 p.m.	Giving the body time to digest improves sleep quality and decreases insulin resistance.	Watch: *Run on Fat*
I only eat eggs that are organic and from pasture-raised chickens.	Chickens are fed chemically sprayed grains, antibiotics, and steroids. They are denied sunlight and restricted to sludging around in stool.	Watch: *Supersize Me* & *Supersize Me 2*
I buy organic fruits and vegetables.	They contain higher levels of antioxidants, fewer pesticides, are closer to the food God made for us, and they are not genetically modified.	Watch: *Genetic Roulette*
I only eat meats that are organic, grass fed, free range, and wild caught.	Animals are fed chemically-treated, GMO foods which are not healthy and will not provide the nutrients you need. They also may pass on residual hormones and antibiotics to us.	Watch: *Food Matters*

CHAPTER 6
REMOVING TOXINS FROM YOUR LIFE

When I first started looking at the ingredients in my personal care products, cleaning products, and foods, I focused on eliminating only four things—pesticides, plastics, preservatives, and parabens. This is a great place to start if you want to decrease the toxic load on your family. That way when you shop, you can approach the ingredients list with knowledge and start replacing items one by one.

Understand that not all toxins are created equal. Some eliminate naturally in poop, pee, sweat, and blood. (There are more professional ways to say that, but it's not nearly as fun.) Some toxins stay in your body until a powerful binder takes them out, and if this doesn't happen, many may pass down to the humans that you incubate. No matter how long toxins stay in your system, they can still cause damage in many ways.

Remember the environmental toxin panel I talked about? I tested myself, before and after detox, and also ran it on my toddler. I valued this resource for two reasons: first, it gave me an idea of my successes, and second, it brought to light some hidden offenders I never would have considered. I recommend this test for all of my ladies wanting to get pregnant; I will provide a resource at the end of the book if you would like to do this. Remember, the EWG study found in cord blood 213 chemicals that the U.S. had banned over thirty years ago? Only passing these chemicals down would cause this.

But ladies, if you feel the burden completely on yourself, check out this study. According to the American Society for Reproductive Medicine, the male partner either solely causes or contributes to infertility in about 40 percent of infertile couples. We're seeing an alarming rise in sperm and semen abnormalities, including lower sperm counts, misshapen sperm, and sperm that cannot swim well. Scientists are now acknowledging that toxins mimic our hormones and wreak havoc on our health.

The Environmental Working Group released a report in 2014 concerning men's health issues and provided a quick list to protect his little swimmers:

- Avoid food in cans or plastic containers.
- Eat organic fruits and vegetables.
- Consult EWG's "Skin Deep Cosmetics Database" for your personal care products.

I would like to add, choose organic, hormone-free meats.

If you need a reason to rope your sperm donor into this journey of preparing your body to grow a human, here it is! Tell them their little swimmers are counting on them to make a few changes too. Note: I refer to *sperm donor* lovingly, whether they are your spouse, partner, or actual sperm donor. For detailed steps on increasing male sperm count, I encourage you to order a copy of *Brighton Baby* by

Roy Dittmann. I have personally used some of this man's passionate and detailed recommendations. Overall, it is an excellent resource.

For this book, I interviewed environmental toxin expert Lara Adler, a speaker at one of Health Centers of The Future's "Live It to Lead It" events. I love the name of our gatherings, as we truly do have to *live* something out before we can *lead* others to change. Lara Adler has conducted an amazing amount of research on toxins and created an online course for learning about toxins in our environment. She designed it specifically for practitioners and health coaches, but it serves as a detailed resource for anyone seeking a deeper understanding of toxins.

I asked if she could help me give people a good starting place for detoxification. Recognizing that every person has different health conditions, different goals, and starting points, we settled on these four priorities: organic food, water, the avoidance of plastics, and the establishment of a healthy mouth–body connection. In other words, clean up your mouth.

Organic Food

I have eaten organic vegetables and fruit for about twenty years as my mom sought to improve our family's health, but I have only eaten organic meats for about ten years. Since then, my social and professional circles primarily contain those who agree with me on the foundational importance of avoiding pesticides as much as possible. Stepping outside my own bubble, I wanted to see what the rest of the world would find if they looked up the facts. I searched for "organic versus non-organic" on YouTube and Google. I found countless videos and papers reporting no significant difference between organic and nonorganic food, except for the price. *Ugh*. I feel it would help to do a little myth busting for you.

Many of the arguments seemed like nothing more than false reporting on bad science, which frankly enraged me. If I had not known the things I know, this information would have quickly misled me, and I would have dropped the whole idea of going organic. Refer back to chapter 2 for the discussion of glyphosate and other pesticides; buying organic is the best solution for avoiding these. Since this factors into preparing your body to grow a human, I want to give you some research to convince you as well as the person who may help you pay for groceries. I persuaded my man to only buy organic meats in part by planning our meals. Instead of cooking an entire pack of chicken for $7.00, I cooked only what we needed. We wasted nothing and stretched $7.00 (vs. $4.00 for nonorganic) over two meals. This may not work in your family, but try to get creative and do the best you can.

In a short, documentary-style video I watched, a family of six in Sweden ran urine tests and found many different pesticides in each of the family members. They then cleared all the nonorganic food out of the family's home, and for one week ate only organic food. At the end of the week, they repeated the urine tests and compared the results. They found drastic decreases in the amounts of pesticides in each family member's body. Now at first that may make you feel warm and fuzzy, like *Okay, I can switch to organic food at any time, and all will be fine.* But remember, certain toxins can do damage as they're passing through your body, even though you're eliminating them. This tells us, "Go organic ASAP."

Every year the Environmental Working Group puts out "Clean Fifteen & the Dirty Dozen," a list of the most important fruits and vegies to buy organic. For example, strawberries and peaches soak up far more pesticides than pineapple or avocado. Check out another food safety tool on whatsonmyfood.org, where you can find pesticide-residue data collected by the USDA with toxicological profiles, in an easily searchable database. For example, you can look up a specific food to find the number of pesticides it contains, and if they are linked to cancer or hormonal issues. The concern doesn't just lie with veggies and fruits; pesticides land in bread and anything else made from a sprayed crop. They have even tested several baby foods for your future use.

One UK report analyzed government data on pesticide residues over a thirteen-year time span. Researchers found that residues had significantly increased over time, and that the frequency of residues in bread had more than doubled over the study's time period, from 28 percent in 2001 to 63 percent in 2013. The number of samples testing positive for multiple residues have also more than doubled in the last seven years.

I found a very disturbing video clip of a popular television show (that shall remain unnamed) with a food scientist dismissing the dangers of pesticides. She explained that because pesticide exposure to humans occurs in only parts per billion, they were completely safe—people should avoid the cost of organic and just by conventional food. This lady is off her rocker if you ask me! Since pesticides are chemicals meant to kill bugs, it is certainly not crazy to think they could damage human tissue as well.

Let's take a look at the effects of one common pesticide. You can view this information on pesticideinfo.org.

Organophosphate insecticides can invade the body through skin, lungs, or digestive system. The intoxication with organophosphate insect killers results in various signs and symptoms reflecting the affection of numerous organs and systems. Organophosphates provoke acute intoxication in humans with general weakness, tremors, headaches, concentration disturbances, abdominal cramps, nausea, vomiting, diarrhea, excessive perspiration, salivation, and lachrymation. In serious cases, respiratory failure and even death may occur. Several weeks after exposure, doctors may diagnose severe neuropathy with sensations of burning and tingling passing to the paralysis of the lower extremities.

Delayed Consequences of Organophosphate Poisoning

> Exposure may lead to cumulative intoxication with unfavorable effects on the nervous system. Researchers find psychological and behavioral changes in humans after the exposure to the organophosphate insecticides. Agricultural organophosphate insecticides may provoke depression and even suicide attempts.
>
> Organophosphate insecticides are associated with short-sightedness and Saku disease. Saku disease is characterized by the optic neuropathy and visual disturbances such as myopia, astigmatism, reduced vision, narrowing of the visual fields, degeneration of ciliary muscle and retina.
>
> Doctors also observed heart effects associated with professional exposure to organophosphate insect killers such as slowing of the heart rate, reduced cardiac output, myocarditis, and heart attacks.

Now while these side effects may seem dramatic, remember the toxic bucket illustration? A conventional apple won't cause sudden death, with a visual like the apple scene in *Snow White*. The primary concern lies in the constant filling of your bucket, the starting levels of your toxic load, and what final addition may tip your bucket over and spill it.

Water

I am sure you remember from elementary science class that water composes the majority of your body and depriving it of adequate amounts will affect its ability to function. Have you ever had a massage while dehydrated, then felt similar symptoms to the flu afterward? The massage released toxins from your tissues, and your body didn't have enough water to flush it out. Water moves toxins out of the body. Stay hydrated as an easy way to assist your built-in detoxification pathways. A professor of mine once said that by the time you get a headache from dehydration, at least five other organ systems are suffering. You can search the internet and find a great pep talk on the benefits of water and increasing your hydration, but I want to dive into the quality of your water. Water can contain many toxins. Because it is so vital to our survival, I'd like to share its connection to improving the environment you plan to grow your baby in!

Consider these water-related tips. For one, do not drink it out of plastic containers. Plastics can leach into your water as it sits in the bottles through packaging, transit, and shelf time at the store. BPA and other plastics are endocrine disruptors that can cause problems with your hormones. Make the easy switch to drinking out of glass or stainless steel daily. If your city provides poor-quality water and you need to buy bottled, try getting a water cooler and a large jug of spring water with much sturdier plastic. The best-case scenario: use a good filter that will ease your mind about what is in your water.

Chlorine added to city water kills bacteria. Although officials claim that trace amounts should not hurt us, they rarely regulate chlorine levels from the standpoint of keeping people healthy. When I lived in Nashville, a hairdresser asked where I swam because I had so much chlorine damage in my hair. I had not been swimming in a pool in over a year. My everyday showers had done the damage. Yikes! Clearly not regulated.

Water often contains another terrible additive: fluoride. Fluoride is so corrosive that it has to be stored in special containers, could eat a hole in concrete, and can dissolve metal. Take note: as fluoride in the water passes through older pipes, it leaches lead into the water, so it also contributes to increased lead levels in our bodies. Holy smokes, why would we put this in our water? Check out the book *The Case Against Fluoride—How Hazardous Waste Ended Up in Our Drinking Water and the Bad Science and Powerful Politics That Keep It There*. Basically, the title lets you know what underlies the fluoridation of our water without even reading it: Yep, you guessed it. Money.

I recommend testing your home water for heavy metals, pesticides, and other chemicals added to or leaching into your supply. A good test kit ranges from $120 on up, but you can find some $20 tests to at least look for lead. I ordered a kit from Doctor's Data and was happy with its thoroughness.

If I were to sum up the water section in one sentence, I would say, *get a good filter and drink water out of glass.*

Purchasing a good filter may seem simple, but with so many choices, expect to do some research. Affordable options exist and are worth the investment. I purchased a Berkey filter for my office with an additional fluoride filter for under $300. If that option extends beyond your immediate budget, you can purchase a personal water bottle that filters fluoride for under $40. Our home provides spring water, so we bought a whole-house Aquasauna filter for around $1100. Or consider Dime Water's filtration option at http://edmonds.revelationhealth.shop.

Avoiding Plastics

Oh, BPA, how you ruin so many things! BPA's primary damage comes from mimicking hormones. God made us, in part, of little chemicals. It is wise to respect the fact that man-made chemicals could interact with and wreak havoc on our intricate hormonal system. I encourage you to learn about the many types of harmful plastics and avoid them whenever possible, but I chose to highlight BPA here.

Many plastics in water bottles, baby bottles, dental fillings and sealants, dental devices, and epoxy resins (used to coat the inside of food and beverage cans) contain BPA or Bisphenol A. I didn't know this until I saw that the label on my can of organic coconut cream read, "BPA-free lining" and I learned more about it. I even found BPA lurking on the lid of disposable coffee cups. Don't panic—just take your own stainless-steel cup to your favorite coffee location! When you want to take it to the next level, brew your own organic coffee (conventional can contain high pesticide levels) at home and avoid any artificial flavorings or sweeteners.

Back to BPA. How does it really affect our bodies? In 2015, the *Hormones and Behavior* journal published a review of previous studies, finding evidence that BPA can interfere with endocrine function involving the hypothalamus and the pituitary gland. That mechanism, in turn, could potentially elicit problems with puberty, ovulation, and fertility. They also added that "the detrimental effects on reproduction may be lifelong and transgenerational."

This is a real struggle my friends, but we are all in it together. Start by removing as many sources of toxins as you can, then let's detox this garbage out of our bodies!

Environmental Toxins Summary

Environmental Toxins - High

Test Name	In Control	Moderate	High	Current Level	Previous Level
Dimethylphosphate (DMP) (mcg/g)	≤5.20	5.21–37.19	≥37.20	95.36	
mono-(2-ethyl-5-hydroxyhexyl) phthalate (MEHHP) (mcg/g)	≤42.00	42.01–168.99	≥169.00	573.88	
Bisphenol A (BPA) (mcg/g)	≤3.20	3.21–10.80	≥10.81	27.16	

Environmental Toxins - Moderate

Test Name	In Control	Moderate	High	Current Level	Previous Level
Glyphosate (mcg/g)	≤0.75	0.76–2.29	≥2.30	1.36	
3-Phenoxybenzoic Acid (3PBA) (mcg/g)	≤0.57	0.58–6.39	≥6.40	3.28	
Tiglylglycine (TG) (mcg/g)	≤0.10	0.11–11.29	≥11.30	5.68	
2-Hydroxyisobutyric Acid (2HIB) (mcg/g)	≤1005.00	1005.01–5789.99	≥5790.00	4566.15	

Remember my son's Environmental Toxins test? Three of his highest numbers fell in the plastics category, so I want to share the report with you. Under the elevated phthalates, it read,

> "These are known as plasticizers, and they're a group of chemicals used to make plastics more flexible and harder to break. They're widely used in cosmetics, adhesives, detergents, lubricating oils, automotive, plastics, and plastic clothes. People are exposed to phthalates by eating contaminated foods, drinking treated water, but also by breathing air that contains phthalate vapors or dusts. Inhaling phthalates can irritate the nose and throat causing coughing, wheezing, headache, dizziness, and nausea. Phthalates have been classified as endocrine disruptors,

which may cause reproductive damage, depressed leukocyte function, and even cancer. Valid exposure has also been associated with diabetes and insulin resistance, breast cancer, obesity, metabolic disorders and immune disorders. Phthalate exposure and adverse child neuro development, including the development of ADHD, autistic behaviors, and lower cognitive and motor development have also been reported."

My friends, I don't know if this gave you goosebumps, but it blew my mind. We've proven that phthalates can cause all of these problems, and yet we still allow them in thousands of products. Did you notice the side effect, "adverse child neurodevelopment"? This refers to the development of a child's nervous system. BPA is clearly not our only nemesis; many other plastics are wreaking havoc on our hormones.

For some people testing can seem scary because we don't know what we will find. I chose to view my son's testing as a great opportunity to find out how his exposure occurred. I could have felt guilty, but I did my best with the information I had at the time. Now my little dude gets to do a little detoxing, and I get to step up my anti-plastics game!

Clean Cookware

My friend's mom was about to fry us up some eggs for breakfast when she held up two skillets and asked, "Would you like Alzheimer's disease or cancer with your eggs?" You might have guessed it: she offered up an aluminum skillet and a nonstick-coated skillet. That was, sadly, actually several years before she received a diagnosis of stage 3 breast cancer. She had heard enough people say that neither skillet option was great, but really didn't know about any other options were. Ten to twenty and even thirty years ago, this information was harder to come by. In fact, as I learn about these toxins and share them with my family, my mom always sighs, "Oh, I wish I could have done better." Let me be the first to say, *No mommy guilt here!* When we know better, we do better. When we do not know, it is just part of the journey. We can give ourselves grace and keep learning.

Your best options? Stainless steel or cast iron. I use my great-grandma's cast iron and stainless-steel pots for everyday use. Even some of the newer skillets that say, "PFOA-free" have a similar compound, simply another version of the PFOAs.

> *No mommy guilt here!* When we know better, we do better. When we do not know, it is just part of the journey. We can give ourselves grace and keep learning.

What is a PFOA, you ask? Perfluorooctanoic acid (PFOA) and perfluorooctane sulfonate (PFOS) are in the family of perfluorinated compounds (PFCs). Humans carry PFCs, and we are finding that they are more damaging than we could have imagined.

PFOA is used in the manufacture of nonstick cookware (e.g., Teflon) and waterproof fabrics (e.g., Gore-Tex). Because of the stability of the chemical, our bodies and the environment have a difficult time breaking them down. Due to this, nearly every human stores detectable levels of PFCs in their blood.

The short story, switch up your cookware ASAP. Because of the direct correlation between PFCs, fertility, and tiny human exposure, I will dive a little deeper for you.

In 2010, the National Collaborating Centre for Environmental Health put out an evidence review, "*Potential Human Health Effects of Perfluorinated Chemicals* (PFCs)," written by Glenys Webster. This review provides excellent resources, so I include here a summary of relevant content.

- To date, associations have been found between PFOS or PFOA levels in the general population and reduced female fertility and sperm quality, reduced birth weight, attention deficit hyperactivity disorder (ADHD), increased total and non-HDL (bad) cholesterol levels, *and changes in thyroid hormone levels*. Some results are inconsistent across studies and further work is needed to confirm these initial findings.

- In a **highly exposed community** living near a chemical plant, PFOS and PFOA have been associated with *preeclampsia (pregnancy-induced hypertension), birth defects* (PFOA only), and increased uric acid levels—a marker of heart disease. Chemical exposures to the developing fetus, infants, and children are the greatest concern; these periods are the most sensitive stages of human development.

(Italics emphasis mine)

Find PFCs here:

- stain, grease, and water repellents
- fast food packaging
- paper plates
- stain-resistant carpets
- carpet cleaning solutions
- windshield washing fluid
- fire-fighting foam
- some adhesives

- cosmetics
- pharmaceuticals
- electronics
- cleaning products
- polishes and waxes
- insecticides
- paints

Okay, that was intense information, but I refuse to sugar-coat it just because it may induce overwhelm. At the end of the day, I will give you the best resources to conquer these challenges, and you can choose to do with them what you want! Enact one simple change at a time, and most importantly—implement the detox solution I give you to pull these inevitable invaders out of your body!

Clean Dentistry

The toxicity of our mouths can dictate the health of our bodies. We know that gut health sets the foundation of our immune system, and our gut–brain connection significantly impacts hormone regulation, but the picture of our health goes much deeper. I interviewed Dr. Caitlin Czezowski for information on the mouth–body connection because dental work dramatically impacted her own journey of healing. Sealants applied to "protect her teeth from cavities" as well as cavitation infections years after wisdom tooth extraction composed a few of many challenges that have played into her adult health. Out of this journey, she birthed *The Dental Detox*, which has helped thousands of women recover their health by creating it. Dr. Caitlin Czezowski practices as a certified functional medicine practitioner and a doctor of chiropractic with extensive training in women's health, pregnancy, and pediatric dental care.

Every tooth in your mouth connects to a meridian system that correlates with specific organs or glands. Every tooth also connects to the lymphatic system. If our mouth bacteria is out of balance, then any biotoxin that accumulates as an infection will dump directly into the lymphatic system and travel throughout the whole body. Root canals and oral surgeries (such as wisdom tooth removal) can leave behind deteriorating tissue that leads to low-grade infections and biotoxins that target the nervous system. If you suspect that you may have this issue, I have resources and protocols to help you recover your health. Again, don't let this overwhelm you!

As we look for sources of toxins, we need to pay careful attention to the dentist we choose for our families. Seeking out a holistic or biological dentist will help you follow some of Dr. Caitlin's recommendations. Silver fillings may be the most obvious toxin after reading this far. However, many sealants contain BPA, which affects estrogen. Before you have any work done, discuss the fluoride rinse treatment with your dentist (standard procedure in most dental offices). Even some of the white composite fillings may contain components incompatible with your system. If your dentist's knowledge is up-to-date, they will be aware of biocompatibility testing.

Here's a summary of good choices for dental health:

- Quality toothpaste (Revitin is our favorite)
- No fluoride treatments
- No sealants
- No amalgam or silver fillings

- No root canals
- Extractions and implants should be performed by a biological dentist.

Okay, Help Me Fix It

I have no doubt that you may feel overwhelmed at this point, especially if you've never heard some of this information on toxins. I get overwhelmed some days, and I know it well enough to teach, coach, and write about it. But if you only take one thing out of this book, I hope you choose the True Cellular Detox program. You may never change your food, water, personal products, and so on. Or you may not want to pursue any testing, but you can at least clean up the toxins in your body and make room for more. *Ha*! For your enjoyment, here is my favorite analogy about detoxifying:

Picture your body like the hall closet—it's great for coats, shoes, extra toilet paper, wrapping paper, garden boots, paper plates, the toaster you still need to take back to the store—the point is, this closet collects *everything*. As you may have guessed in this cute little analogy, all the "stuff" represents toxins. So, what if you never cleaned the closet? Not ever! One day the door would never shut, and everything would spill out. (I always picture the main character in the movie *27 Dresses* with her closet exploding with bridesmaids' dresses.) But just like the toxic bucket overflowing—everything falling out of the closet represents symptoms. So what's a girl to do? *Clean out your closet!* Especially before you have a baby! Oh, and maybe stop putting so much garbage in the closet too! Hint hint: R1, removing the source.

Another important thought about the closet, AKA our bodies. Even if you overhauled it a year or two ago, you will still periodically need to clean it out again. For this reason,

I love coaching people through the True Cellular Detox program. I not only help them in the moment, I give them tools that they and their families can use for the rest of their lives. Let's face it, our world is not going to get any less toxic, so we need to arm ourselves with the right weapons and strategies to take the enemy out!

> Our world is not going to get any less toxic, so we need to arm ourselves with the right weapons and strategies to take the enemy out!

True Cellular Detox Solution

Detox as a word can take on many implications. As I use it here, it means detoxing your body in the proper order, getting to the cellular level, and most importantly, reaching the brain and deeper tissues to remove the actual cause of dysfunction. This means that a ten-day cleanse will not cut it. A colon or liver detox alone will not achieve your goals. You have to support and clean out your liver, kidneys, gut, and lymph before you start detoxing, otherwise the dislodged toxins will have no way out of your body. You then must detox the cells and tissues before using products that cross the blood–brain barrier. This creates a gradient to pull the heavy metals and biotoxins from the brain.

Dr. Pompa created this program out of necessity after helping tens of thousands of people regain their health. You will need multiple supplements and nutraceuticals to support the body, but instead of having thirty-two bottles along with confusion, Dr. Pompa provided nicely organized packets with videos with specific detoxing instructions. Now that is a busy woman's dream!

We have talked about hundreds of chemicals that negatively impact your health. It is nearly impossible to avoid all of them. Navigating the True Cellular Detox program will arm you with confidence that you are binding as many of these toxins as possible, *safely*! It repairs the detoxification pathways God built into you, so you can more efficiently eliminate daily toxins as you go on to grow a healthy human.

Just take a moment and imagine your life and how you would feel if all of your organs had the ability to function at a higher level. Imagine how you would sleep better. How you would show up better for your loved ones. How your energy would improve and how you would then be able to fulfill your purpose and goals for this life. After all, we only get one of those . . .

HealthyHumanDetox.com to get started!

CHAPTER 7
THE MOST IMPORTANT THING

When trying to do something, and do it well, do you make a list of all you need to accomplish, then start checking off the boxes? The process of preparing your body to grow a human might feel just like that! There are many important things to do, and the order in which you do them is also important. It's easy to become overwhelmed by a desire to understand and put everything into action we have talked about. You might even wrestle with a little bit of guilt, knowing the amount of toxicity you may have passed on to your children. I want you to remember that you cannot change what you knew, so do not play the "what-if game." That won't do anything but hold your thoughts in a negative pattern. At my practice, we detox kids as young as twelve months old all the time. Give yourself grace. Move forward with a plan for the next time.

We have not discussed perhaps the most important preparation for pregnancy. This is a hard one for me and all of my friends who like to check off the boxes. It's also vital, whether you are hoping to have your first pregnancy or your fourteenth.

Interestingly, this is the last chapter I wrote in this book. I could not write it until I gave my husband the green light to make a baby. For a long while, I felt like I needed to check off more boxes. Finally, though, the pieces fell into place when I interviewed a good friend of mine, Melinda McCoy, who is a midwife. VeritasBirth.com is her website with some wonderful resources and support. I was excited to interview her because who knows better than a midwife how to ready a woman for pregnancy? She catches babies all the time, has years and years of experience helping women from a wide variety of backgrounds, lifestyles, and nutritional habits. I knew that she, of all people, could prioritize the most important tasks for preparing to grow a human. She has seen all kinds of women from all walks of life grow and deliver tiny humans. I asked her many, many questions, and amazingly she didn't tell me how many grams of protein or pounds of dark, leafy greens a woman should eat. She simply said to make sure I was cultivating joy and gratitude. Joy and gratitude.

If you're like me, you're probably thinking, *What? Joy and gratitude—that's it?* It gave me pause at first, too, but the more I pondered it, the more it made perfect sense. Joy. Gratitude. These are not just words on a page. They represent genuine states of being in which humans—at all stages and ages—thrive and grow and find purpose. The emotions of joy and gratitude vibrate at 540 hertz. Every organ system in our body operates on a different frequency. When we change our mindset and change our emotions, it literally affects our physiology.

Whether you've checked off all the boxes, incorporated the healing strategies, done the detox or removed the toxins from your home or not, at the end of the day, it truly counts most to have joy and gratitude. What does that mean? I think it will look different for everyone. I know many people benefit from keeping a gratitude journal that they write in daily. I am thankful that I am a woman and that I get to create the bond that I share with my children. I am thankful that in each step of my journey God will provide the resources I need for that season. We can teach our children gratefulness, and when we live in a state of gratitude, joy seems to come naturally.

I find that I have to repeatedly put down my mental checklist, but there is such peace in letting go that it's worth it. This serves as one of the best tools for toning down my stress. It helps me shut down my sympathetic nervous system in favor of a parasympathetic mode, where I can rest and heal. At the end of the day, some of us find security in trying to control things. We find true peace, however, in letting go and trusting our body and the way that God made it.

> We find true peace in letting go and trusting our body and the way that God made it.

The fact that I can say these words is an amazing testimony to all I've learned. I had a truly hard journey with my first son. As I worked through some of the emotional difficulty, I realized that I had lost trust in my own body because of a very difficult birth process. I had changed the way I viewed birth, changed the way I thought about my own body. When I realized that, I faced it head on. I now have affirmations about getting pregnant, carrying a baby, and having a safe and healthy delivery. No matter the journey, I know I can always change my mindset.

And above all, you deserve to be well.

Starting Your Journey

Building your own timeline is one of the most important parts of preparing your body to grow a human. A timeline has a beginning, a middle, and an end goal (to birth a healthy human). When you set these goals, keep in mind that good health is a journey. Whether you're eliminating toxins, adopting new healthy habits, or doing a bit of everything, those changes will take time to understand, implement, and maintain. It might take a lifetime to push some toxins out of our body. When faced with that sobering reality, getting started can seem a little daunting. For me, creating a timeline saved my sanity!

I suggest you start with the quiz in Chapter 4, move forward with some testing, and implement the True Cellular Detox program (find a link in Resources for the mama-to-be, chapter 5) for three to twelve months. At the same time, work on removing toxins from your home and repairing your health foundation with the strategies I gave you. Sticking to the timeline and waiting for the right timing may prove one of the hardest parts of this journey. It may feel taxing when you're ready to start a family, but you know it's best to wait. For me, it was maddening and frustrating. I had to dig deep in my soul for what I really wanted, but my best insight came from building my timeline and sitting down to do some serious praying.

I believe with 100 percent of my being that God wants the best for us and will intentionally set his care over us. He has great hope and blessed futures planned for all of us (Jeremiah 29:11). I also believe he gives us the resources we need exactly when we need them. Maybe you've already had several children, you are ready to have a baby tomorrow, or are looking three to four years out. No matter where you are on the journey, you have choice. You get to decide the strategies you'll implement, how deep you'll go, and how much time you will take. I had my first child at age thirty-five. I'm sure I would have recovered faster at twenty-five, but I owned a healthier body in my thirties. I was more emotionally capable and it was, frankly, the right time for me. Cheers to having my second child at thirty-eight!

I mentioned that you choose. You must give yourself grace and understand that many factors play into shaping the perfect timeline. Consider your own expectations as well as the expectations of spouses and families. At the end of the day, however, knowing that you did everything in your power to grow the healthiest human possible will give you great peace and satisfaction. Just keep in mind that your power has limits and chances are you will not be able to do everything in this book—and that's okay. God has created us to bear children and has built in mechanisms to protect that baby.

When you finally decide to give your man the green light, let go of all the little things. If you start falling back into worry mode, you won't move forward and may stall your timeline. If you need to, refer back to Emotional Tools in chapter 5. My best advice? Give it all up and ask Jesus to take the wheel!

A Note for When You Do Get Pregnant

When people get a positive pregnancy test, they schedule an appointment with their doctor or midwife, so I want to help set your expectations. First, research topics on your own, then hire a doctor or midwife who supports your beliefs. This might sound like a no-brainer, but your birth experience will be such an emotional experience that it could potentially make or break your first few weeks as a new parent. By *break* I mean break your heart. Let me challenge you to watch *Why Not Home*, an excellent documentary, and if you have the stomach for some live births, an older one called *The Business of Being Born*. (If you don't have the stomach for live births, try watching it anyway to really know what to expect.)

When you find out you're pregnant, find a tribe. We are so overstimulated and overwhelmed with activities, it can be difficult to connect with like-minded women going through a similar life stage. On the other hand, great opportunity exists for connection through online platforms. Only time holds us back. I believe we should do whatever it takes to find community. My community helped me keep my sanity when things got hard.

Have you ever noticed the silent bond between mothers? When you start showing that baby bump, women everywhere open up and share some of the most intimate experiences of pregnancy. Multiple times in a checkout line, restaurant, or store, a woman would notice my bump and begin a trip down memory lane sharing good things, sad things, maybe a piece of advice for the new mama. It is so beautiful to see how deeply ingrained your birth story will be, so cheers to feeling prepared and confident in your body, and may God bless your mind, body, and spirit as you begin this journey of growing a tiny, healthy human!

RESOURCES FOR THE MAMA-TO-BE

I Am Ready to Detox: www.HealthyHumanDetox.com

Testing Recap
Hormone Testing—Dutch dried-urine tests
Thyroid—blood draw (see the Thyroid section for specifics)
Heavy Metals—Doctor's Data provoked-urine challenge
Environmental Toxins—Vibrant America Environmental Toxins test
Inflammation—Meta-Oxy urine test in a TCD practitioner's office

Safe Personal Products
Think Dirty App: https://www.ewg.org/skindeep/

Pregnancy and Pediatric Research and Wellness Articles
www.icpa4kids.org

Webster Technique
https://icpa4kids.com/training/webster-certification/webster-technique/

Glyphosate Research
Stephanie Seneff's Home Page (mit.edu)

Vaccine Information
www.vaccineu.com
www.ChildrensHealthDefence.org
www.1986theact.com

Lymph-Pumping Download
www.notmeds.com
www.thetruewellnesscenter.com

Pure Form Omega
https://revelationhealth.com/products/pureform-omega-natural-120-capsules?_pos=1&_sid=0ca69ae29&_ss=r&afmc=d7&utm_campaign=d7&utm_source=leaddyno&utm_medium=affiliate

Biological Dentist Database
www.IAOMT.org
www.IABDM.org

Prenatal Supplements
www.allisonbonham.juiceplus.com
https://revelationhealth.com/pages/edmonds?afmc=edmonds

Craniosacral Therapists Near You
https://www.iahp.com/pages/search/index.php

Free Tapping Manual
https://eftinternational.org/wp-content/uploads/EFT-International-Free-Tapping-Manual.pdf

Birth Information
www.VeritasBirth.com

BIBLIOGRAPHY

Chapter 1

"Update on Overall Prevalence of Major Birth Defects." Cited in "Data &Statistics on Birth Defects," Centers for Disease Control. MMWR Weekly. January 10, 2008. https://www.cdc.gov/ncbddd/birthdefects/data.html.

"Data and Statistics on Autism Spectrum Disorder." CDC, September 25, 2020. https://www.cdc.gov/ncbddd/autism/data.html.

"Childhood Cancer: Statistics" ASCO Journals, Cancer.net. January 1, 2021. www.cancer.net/cancer-types/childhood-cancer/statistics.

"Data & Statistics on Birth Defects," CDC.gov, https://www.cdc.gov/ncbddd/birthdefects/data.html.

Houlihan, Jane, Timothy Kropp, PhD, Richard Wiles, Sean Gray, Chris Campbell. "Body Burden: The Pollution in Newborns," Environmental Working Group. July 14, 2005. https://www.ewg.org/research/body-burden-pollution-newborns.

Columbia University School of Public Health, 95 percent of cancer is caused by diet and the environment. "Cancer is a Preventable Disease that Requires Major Lifestyle Changes", https://www.ncbi.nlm.nih.gov/pmc/articles/PMC2515569/

Cook, Ken. "10 Americans," by Environmental Working Group, You Tube. July 23, 2012, Video, 22:26. https://youtu.be/0-kc3AIM_LU.

Costello, M. F., M. L. Misso, A. Balen, J. Boyle, L. Devoto, R. M. Garad, R. Hart, et al. "Evidence summaries and recommendations from the international evidence-based guideline for the assessment and management of polycystic ovary syndrome: assessment and treatment of infertility." *Human Open Reproduction.* January 4, 2019. doi: 10.1093/hropen/hoy021.

García-Ibañez, Paula, Lucía Yepes-Molina, Antonio J. Ruiz-Alcaraz, María Martínez-Esparza, Diego A. Moreno, Micaela Carvajal, and Pilar García-Peñarrubia. "Brassica Bioactives Could Ameliorate the Chronic Inflammatory Condition of Endometriosis." *International Journal of Molecular Sciences* 21, no. 24 (December 10, 2020): 9397. doi: 10.3390/ijms21249397.

Chapter 2

"Environment, not genes, dictates human immune variation, study finds." Science Daily. January 15, 2015. www.sciencedaily.com/releases/2015/01/150115134715.htm.

"Data and Statistics on Autism Spectrum Disorder." CDC.gov, https://www.cdc.gov/ncbddd/autism/data.html.

"One in Three Kids Will Develop Diabetes" WebMD, June 16, 2003. https://www.webmd.com/diabetes/news/20030616/one-in-three-kids-will-develop-diabetes.

"Facts & Figures 2021 Reports Another Record-Breaking 1-Year Drop in Cancer Deaths," Cancer.org, January 12, 2021. https://www.cancer.org/latest-news/facts-and-figures-2021.html.

Warner, Jennifer. "Baby Boomers May Outlive Their Kids." WebMD, April 9, 2010. https://www.webmd.com/children/news/20100409/baby-boomers-may-outlive-their-kids.

Zhang, Luoping, Iemaan Rana, Rachel M.Shaffer, EmanuelaTaioli, Lianne Sheppard. "Exposure to glyphosate-based herbicides and risk for non-Hodgkin lymphoma: A meta-analysis and supporting evidence. *Mutation Research* Reviews in Mutation Research 781, (July–September 2019): 186–206. ScienceDirect. https://www.sciencedirect.com/science/article/abs/pii/S1383574218300887.

Seneff, Stephanie, and Rachel F. Orlando. Glyphosate Substitution for Glycine During Protein Synthesis as a Causal Factor in Mesoamerican Nephropathy." *Environmental and Analytical Toxicology* 8, no. 1 (2018): Hilaris. DOI: 10.4172/2161-0525.10005 41.

Seneff, Stephanie, Nicholas J. Causton, Gregory L. Nigh, Gerald Koenig, and Dette Avalon. "Can glyphosate's disruption of the gut microbiome and induction of sulfate deficiency explain the epidemic in gout and associated diseases in the industrialized world?" *Journal of Biological Physics and Chemistry* 17, (2017): 53–76. http://www.amsi.ge/jbpc/21717/04SE17A.pdf.

Seneff, Stephanie. MIT Homepage. https://people.csail.mit.edu/seneff.

Dalsager, Louise et al. "Maternal urinary concentrations of pyrethroid and chlorpyrifos metabolites and attention deficit hyperactivity disorder (ADHD) symptoms in 2-4-year-old children from the Odense Child Cohort."

Environmental Research. Vol. 176 (2019): 108533. DOI: 10.1016/j.envres.2019.108533

Alengebawy, Ahmed, Sara Taha Abdelkhalek, Sundas Rana Qureshi, and Man-Qun Wang. "Heavy Metals and Pesticides Toxicity in Agricultural Soil and Plants: Ecological Risks and Human Health Implications." *Toxics* 9, no. 3 (Feb. 2021): doi:10.3390/toxics9030042.

"Obama signs 'Monsanto Protection Act' written by Monsanto-sponsored senator." *RT Question More*. March 8, 2013. https://www.rt.com/usa/monsanto-bill-blunt-agriculture-006/.

Gasnier, Céline, Coralie Dumont, Nora Benachour, Emilie Clair, Marie-Christine Chagnon, and Gilles-Eric Séralini. "Glyphosate-based herbicides are toxic and endocrine disruptors in human cell lines." *Toxicology*. 262, no. 3 (August 21, 2009): 184–191. https://www.sciencedirect.com/science/article/pii/S0300483X09003047

Marques, Ana, Sofia Guilherme, Isabel Gaivão, Maria Ana Santos, and Mário Pacheco. "Progression of DNA damage induced by a glyphosate-based herbicide in fish (*Anguilla anguilla*) upon exposure and post-exposure periods — Insights into the mechanisms of genotoxicity and DNA repair." *Comparative Biochemistry and Physiology Part C: Toxicology & Pharmacology*. 166 (November 2014): 126–133. ScienceDirecct. https://doi.org/10.1016/j.cbpc.2014.07.009.

Rees, Nicholas and Richard Fuller. "The Toxic Truth: Children's Exposure to Lead Pollution Undermines a Generation of Future Potential." UNICEF and Pure Earth. https://www.unicef.org/sites/default/files/2020-07/The-toxic-truth-children%E2%80%99s-exposure-to-lead-pollution-2020.pdf.

Ericson, Bret, Jack Caravanos, Kevin Chatham-Stephens, Philip Landrigan, and Richard Fuller. "Approaches to

Systematic Assessment of Environmental Exposures Posed at Hazardous Waste Sites in the Developing World: The Toxic Sites Identification Program." *Environmental Monitoring and Assessment* 185, no. 2 (2013): 1755–1766. https://doi.org/10.1007/s10661-012-2665-2.

ATSDR. Environmental Health and Medicine. "Case Studies in Environmental Medicine: Lead Toxicity: Clinical Assessment—Signs and Symptoms." Last reviewed July 2, 2019. https://www.atsdr.cdc.gov/csem/leadtoxicity/signs_and_symptoms.html.

Chen, Chi et al. "Associations of blood lead levels with reproductive hormone levels in men and postmenopausal women: Results from the SPECT-China Study." *Scientific Reports* 6 (Nov 29, 2016). PMC. doi:10.1038/srep37809.

Darryl Fears. "It's not just Flint. Lead taints water across the U.S., EPA records show." *The Washington Post*, March 16, 2017. https://www.washingtonpost.com/news/energy-environment/wp/2016/03/17/its-not-just-flint-lead-taints-water-across-the-u-s-the-epa-says/.

"Shock Report: 18 Cities in Pennsylvania Have Higher Lead Exposure Than Flint" Sept 30, 2016. Martin Water. https://nicmarwater.com/blog/shock-report-18-cities-in-pennsylvania-have-higher-lead-exposure-than-flint/.

U.S. FDA. "Limiting Lead in Lipstick and Other Cosmetics." August 24, 2020. https://www.niehs.nih.gov/health/topics/agents/lead/index.cfm

Ziff, Sam, and Michael F. *Dentistry Without Mercury.* ([city, publ.,] 2014).

Oskarsson, A. A. Schültz, S. Skerfving, I.P. Hallén, B. Ohlin, and B.J. Lagerkvist. "Total and inorganic mercury in breast milk in relation to fish consumption and amalgam in lactating women." *Archives of Environmental Health* 51. No. 3 (1996): 234–41. doi:

10.1080/00039896.1996.9936021. PMID: 8687245. https://pubmed.ncbi.nlm.nih.gov/8687245/.

L. da Costa, Sérgio. "Breast-Milk Mercury Concentrations and Amalgam Surface in Mothers from Brasília, Brazil." *Biological Trace Element Research* 106, no. 2 (Sept 2005): 145–51. PubMed. DOI:10.1385/BTER:106:2:145.

Genchi, Giuseppe, G. Genchi, M. S. Sinicropi, A. Carocci, G. Lauria, and A. Catalano. "Mercury Exposure and Heart Diseases." *International Journal of Environmental Research and Public Health* 14, no. 1 (Jan. 12, 2017): 74. PubMed. doi:10.3390/ijerph14010074.

Myers, Iris. "5 Things To Avoid in Your Personal Care Products If You're Pregnant or Trying To Get Pregnant." October 13, 2020. EWG. https://www.ewg.org/news-insights/news/5-things-avoid-your-personal-care-products-if-youre-pregnant-or-trying-get.

"Historical Advisories Where You Live" EPA.gov, https://fishadvisoryonline.epa.gov/General.aspx

Nissen, Thomas. "Mercury Poisoning Toxicity: An In-depth Report on the Effects of Mercury Poisoning Toxicity." eventbetterhealth.com. https://www.evenbetterhealth.com/heavy-metal-poisoning-mercury.asp.

"Heavy Metal." *Science Direct.* https://www.sciencedirect.com/topics/chemistry/heavy-metal

"National Childhood Vaccine Injury Act of 1986," Congress.gov, https://www.congress.gov/bill/99th-congress/house-bill/5546

"Toxic Metals," OSHA.gov, https://www.osha.gov/toxic-metals

Shoemaker, Ritchie C. Judith M. Rash, and Elliott W. Simon. "Sick Building Syndrome in Water Damaged Buildings: Generalization of the Chronic Biotoxin-Associated

Illness Paradigm to Indoor Toxigenic Fungi." Center for Research on Biotoxin Associated Illnesses. https://www.survivingmold.com/docs/Resources/Shoemaker%20Papers/Johanning_book_5_06.pdf.

Duke University. *Ciphers.* "Part 2: What is epigenetics, and what does it mean for CIPHERS?" June 6, 2019. https://sites.duke.edu/ciphers/2019/06/06/part-2-what-is-epigenetics-and-what-does-it-mean-for-ciphers/.

Seneff, Stephanie, Davidson, R.M., and Liu, J. "Empirical Data Confirm Autism Symptoms Related to Aluminum and Acetaminophen Exposure." *Entropy* 2012, no. 14, 2227-2253. https://doi.org/10.3390/e14112227.

Chapter 3

Mayo Clinic. "Preconception planning: Is your body ready for pregnancy?" December 12, 2020. https://www.mayoclinic.org/healthy-lifestyle/getting-pregnant/in-depth/preconception/art-20046664.

Shkodzik, Kate. "10 Essential Things to Do Before Getting Pregnant." Updated on August 24, 2020. Flo. https://flo.health/getting-pregnant/10-essential-things-to-do-before-getting-pregnant.

American Thyroid Association. "Hypothyroidism in Pregnancy." https://www.thyroid.org/hypothyroidism-in-pregnancy/.

Pompa, Dan. "Back to the Basics: The 5R's of True Cellular Detox and Healing." August 15, 2014. https://drpompa.com/cellular-detox.

Stoiber, Tasha. "What Are Parabens, and Why Don't They Belong in Cosmetics?" *Environmental Working Group.* April 9, 2019. https://www.ewg.org/what-are-parabens.

Lipton, Bruce. "Bruce Lipton on Mastering Your Destiny." *Awaken*. https://awaken.com/2020/08/nde-my-experience-in-coma.

Lipton, Bruce H. Homepage. www.brucelipton.com.

"Tackling the burden of chronic diseases in the USA." *The Lancet*. Volume 73. January 17, 2009. https://www.thelancet.com/action/showPdf?pii=S0140-6736%2809%2960048-9.

"Chronic Diseases in America." *National Center for Chronic Disease Prevention and Health Promotion*. January 12, 2021. https://www.cdc.gov/chronicdisease/resources/infographic/chronic-diseases.htm.

Marchese, Marianne. "Parabens and Breast Cancer." *Natural Medicine Journal*. Vol. 2, no. 10. October 2010.

Morgan, Daniel. "Methylation Polymorphisms Are More Complicated Than MTHFR." The Center for Integrative Wellness. https://naturopathic.doctor/methylation-polymorphisms-are-more-complicated-than-mthfr/.

U.S. National Library of Medicine. MTHFR gene. https://medlineplus.gov/genetics/gene/mthfr/. Kircheimer, Sid. "Year 2000 Babies High Risk for Diabetes." WebMD. October 7, 2003. https://www.webmd.com/diabetes/news/20031007/year-2000-babies-high-risk-for-diabetes#.

Chapter 5

Anthon, Kiara and Timothy J. Legg. "EFT Tapping." *Healthline*. https://www.healthline.com/health/eft-tapping#technique. September 18, 2018.

Blakeway, Jill. "Acupuncture During Pregnancy - Acupuncture Pregnancy." *The Yinova Center*. 21 July 2020, www.yinovacenter.com/blog/acupuncture-during-pregnancy-2.

Zhu J, Arsovska B, Kozovska K. Acupuncture Treatment for Fertility. *Open Access Maced J Med Sci.* 2018;6(9):1685-1687. September 19, 018. doi:10.3889/oamjms.2018.379.

Hunter, Brenda. *The Power of Mother Love: Strengthening the Bond Between You and Your Child.* (Colorado Springs, CO: WaterBrook Press, 1999).

Chapter 6

"Clean Fifteen: EWG's 2021 Shopper's Guide to Pesticides in Produce." Environmental Working Group. https://www.ewg.org/foodnews/clean-fifteen.php.

Pesticide Action Network of North America. "Pesticides: A Public Problem." WhatsOnMyFood.org.

Pesticide Info. Pesticide Action Network. www.pesticideinfo.org.

"Loaf-threatening: More than half of British breads contain 'toxic' pesticides," *RT Question More.* July 17, 2014. https://www.rt.com/uk/173476-pesticide-toxic-uk-poison.

Machtinger, Ronit, Catherine M H Combelles, Stacey A Missmer, Katharine F Correia, Paige Williams, Russ Hauser, Catherine Racowsky. "Bisphenol-A and human oocyte maturation in vitro," *Human Reproduction.* Volume 28, Issue 10, October 2013, Pages 2735–2745, doi.org/10.1093/humrep/det312.

Wolstenholme, Jennifer T. Emilie F. Rissman, and Jessica J. Connelly.. "The role of Bisphenol A in shaping the brain, epigenome and behavior," *Hormones and Behavior.* Volume 59, Issue 3, March 2011, Pages 296-305. doi: 10.1016/j.yhbeh.2010.10.001

Brazier, Yvette and Suzanne Flack. "How does bisphenol A affect health?". *Medical News Today.* May 25, 2017. https://www.medicalnewstoday.com/articles/221205.

Webster, Glenys. "Potential human health effects of perfluorinated chemicals (PFCs)," *National Collaborating Centre for Environmental Health*. October 2010. https://www.ncceh.ca/sites/default/files/Health_effects_PFCs_Oct_2010.pdf.

Gore, Andrea C, Krittika Krishnan, Michael P Reilly. "Endocrine-disrupting chemicals: Effects on neuroendocrine systems and the neurobiology of social behavior," *Hormones and Behavior*. Volume 111, May 2019, Pages 7-22. doi: 10.1016/j.yhbeh.2018.11.006.

Krieg, Sacha A., Lora K. Shahine, Ruth B. Lathi. "Environmental exposure to endocrine-disrupting chemicals and miscarriage." *Fertility and Sterility*. Volume 106, Issue 4, P941-947, September 15, 2016. doi.org/10.1016/j.fertnstert.2016.06.043.

* * *

ABOUT THE AUTHOR

Allison Edmonds, DC, is committed to empowering women to take control of their health. She speaks regularly about fasting, detoxification, and other practices that equip people to reclaim their health. Allison is particularly passionate about reaching young women with information to empower them to take responsibility for their wellness and the health of their unborn children.

Suffering from allergies, asthma, and headaches as a child, Allison became interested in how the body works. Her passion only grew with time, and she became a staunch advocate for mothers and babies. Allison earned a bachelor's degree in exercise science from the University of Cincinnati, a doctorate in chiropractic, and a license in physical therapy from Life University. She is a certified Health Centers of the Future practitioner with expertise in detoxification and cellular healing.

Allison and her husband, Dan, own Freedom Family Chiropractic where they take a fresh, innovative approach to spinal correction by incorporating nutrition, exercise, and detoxification into their practice.

Allison lives in Dayton, Ohio, with her husband and son. You can connect with her at DrAllisonEdmonds.com.

When you're not ready for the book to end...

JOIN OUR COMMUNITY

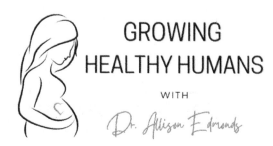

Today's statistics are staggering:

- » Babies are being born with 287 chemicals in their tiny bodies.
- » 1 in 4 children are being diagnosed with a mental health condition.
- » 1 in 3 children born after 2000 will have diabetes.
- » Toxins are driving inflammation, causing diseases and even cancer in children.
- » The number of children diagnosed with autism is currently increasing exponentially.

Your children's health is challenged like never before. The good news is your body=baby's environment, so there *is* something you can do to give your child a healthier start.

In the Growing Healthy Humans community, we will coach families like yours through a process to remove the environmental toxins and inflammation that exist at the cellular level. We will show you the healthy and natural pathway to being able to confidently conceive.

We want to help you establish a better foundation for your child's health so you can grow a healthy, happy family.

GrowingHealthyHumans.com

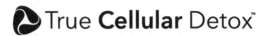

90 Days of 1-on-1 Detox Coaching
to Remove Toxic Metals and Create a Healthy Human

SIGN UP TODAY AND RECEIVE THE FOLLOWING:

- ✓ 90 days of supplement information and instructions
- ✓ Free toxicity testing to measure your progress (4 test kits included)
- ✓ 20+ hours of detox training
- ✓ 130+ cellular healing recipes
- ✓ 90-day meal plan with grocery lists
- ✓ 30 delicious smoothie recipes

- ✓ Monthly calls with your certified True Cellular Detox™ coach
- ✓ Strategies such as intermittent fasting, ketosis, and diet variation
- ✓ FAQ board, email, and online support
- ✓ Burst training benefits
- ✓ De-bunking fat burning myths
- ✓ Mindset training

"Thanks to True Cellular Detox™, I have been able to start eating food again. I feel blessed that I have been led to this program, which has transformed my life. I have great things happening and plan to repeat the program until I have optimal health, which I have never had since birth. There is new hope thanks to this gift! " — *Sharon S.*

Reserve your spot today at
HealthyHumanDetox.com

NOT JUST ANOTHER BORING NUTRITION TALK!

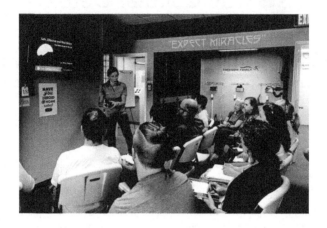

Our children are sicker than ever. Studies show:
- −1 in 4 pregnancies result in miscarriage.
- −1 in 8 couples are unable to conceive.
- −Babies are being born with 287 chemicals in their bodies.

People need real answers regarding these life-altering choices, not boring lectures. Provide your audiences with engaging, energetic revelations regarding these relevant topics, providing hope and strategies they can use.

Dr. Allison Edmonds of Freedom Health Center will tailor her talk to your audience. Her primary topics include:

> **How to Prepare Your Body for a Healthy Human**
> **Toxins and How to Detox at a Cellular Level**
> **Stress, Adrenals, and Hormones**

DrAllisonEdmonds.com/Speaking

Preparing for your healthy human may be overwhelming.

Dr. Allison can help.

Get answers to your questions and help to map out your timeline of detoxing and healing before you conceive.

Dr. Allison will look at your complete patient history and review any previous testing or blood work that you may have available.

Visit
PregnancyPrepChecklist.com
today and begin *your* journey
toward growing a healthy human!

Made in the USA
Monee, IL
28 October 2021